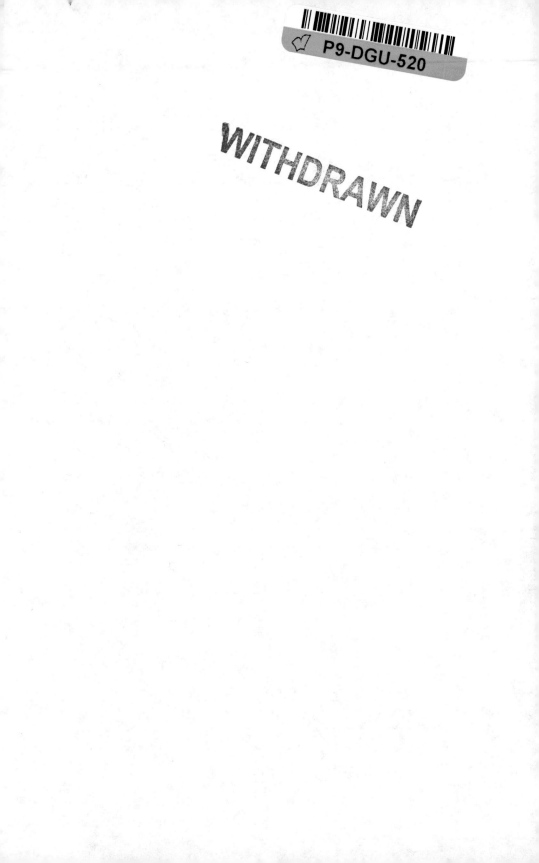

EMERGENCY
FIRST AID

For Your Dog

Tamara S. Shearer, D.V.M.
Edited by Stanford Apseloff

EMERGENCY
FIRST AID

For Your Dog

Tamara S. Shearer, D.V.M.
Edited by Stanford Apseloff

OHIO DISTINCTIVE PUBLISHING
Columbus, Ohio 1996

Published by Ohio Distinctive Publishing, Inc.
6500 Fiesta Drive, Columbus OH 43235
www.ohio-distinctive.com

Printed in the United States of America.

98   8 7

Illustrated by Claudia Beth Sheets

ISBN: 0-9647934-2-3

Library of Congress Catalog Card Number: 96-67366

This book is dedicated to my parents,
my patients
and
dogs everywhere.

Special thanks to Stan and Azaria

ABOUT THE AUTHOR

Dr. Tamara Shearer owns and operates a small-animal veterinary practice in Columbus, Ohio and teaches a dog and cat first-aid course. She is on the Board of Directors of the Columbus Veterinary Emergency Service and is a member of the Citizens for Humane Action Animal Shelter, the American Veterinary Medical Association and the Ohio Veterinary Medical Association. Dr. Shearer has appeared as a veterinary medical advisor on local television and is a university guest lecturer and guest practitioner. Dr. Shearer has a Doctor of Veterinary Medicine degree from The Ohio State University College of Veterinary Medicine and is licensed to practice veterinary medicine in Ohio and California. She is one of the few veterinarians who still make house calls. Dr. Shearer owns four dogs.

TABLE OF CONTENTS

PART 4 - POISON BASICS

General Procedures / 182
List of Common Poisons / 183

PART 5 - POISONOUS PLANTS

Introduction to Poisonous Plants / 186
Poisonous Plants (Listed Alphabetically) / 187
Plants that Cause Skin Irritation / 235
Nonpoisonous Plants / 236

PART 6 - OTHER POISONS

Other Poisons (Listed Alphabetically) / 238

PART 7 - DISEASES THAT CAN BECOME EMERGENCIES

General Information / 256
Dental Disease / 257
Infections and Fever / 258
Cancers / 259
Long-Term Illnesses / 260
Skin Irritations / 261
Soft Stools/Diarrhea / 262
Intestinal Parasites / 264
External Parasites (Listed Alphabetically) / 265

PART 8 - MISCELLANEOUS

APPENDICES

BIBLIOGRAPHY / 297

INDEX / 299

PART 1

—

GETTING STARTED

SPECIAL COMMENTS

This book is a first-aid guide for common emergencies. It is meant to be used as an aid when immediate veterinary care is unavailable. This book should not be used as a substitute for veterinary care. Because your veterinarian will be able to advise you best based on the particular circumstances of your dog's emergency, you should contact your veterinarian at the earliest possible moment, preferably before initiating any nonessential treatment.

INTRODUCTION

It was New Year's Eve, and the Andersons were enjoying the night's festivities, as was Bogart, the family canine. Bogart feasted on the box of chocolates that had been carefully wrapped and placed under the tree. By the time someone noticed, the chocolates were gone and Bogart looked distressed.

This book is designed to teach dog owners, like the Andersons, how to tend to their pet's medical emergencies until they can get professional veterinary assistance. By using the emergency first-aid guidance provided by this book, you can learn to recognize a medical emergency and treat it appropriately.

This book will discuss how to handle the injured or sick dog, how to make a first-aid kit, how to assess an emergency situation, and how to treat your pet during a crisis. This book provides instruction for treating a host of problems ranging from minor ailments to severe situations, including bite wounds, poisoning and being hit by a car.

PREVENTION

The best way to remedy an emergency is to prevent it from happening. By recognizing potential hazards before they occur, you may save your dog's life. Dogs are curious by nature and are adept at finding trouble. Because of the number of hazards outdoors, dogs should, ideally, be confined to the house or kept in a secured yard. Dogs that are permitted to roam outdoors can explore dangerous places, and when they do get into trouble, you might not be there to help. Also, with unconfined dogs it is difficult to monitor attitude, appetite, toilet habits and other behavior for signs of illness; many seriously ill or injured dogs that are not confined seek out hiding places and often die.

Even when dogs are kept mostly inside or in a secured yard, they are often masters of escape. Therefore, all dogs should be provided with an identification tag. The tag should include the owner's name, address, and telephone number on one side and the veterinarian's name, address and telephone number on the opposite side. Proper identification is important in facilitating treatment. If a pet is away from its home and an illness or injury occurs, the owner can be identified and notified of the situation. The identification tag should directly adhere to the pet's collar and should not be left dangling. A dangling tag can become stuck in and on various objects and pose some risk. (However, any identification is better than none.) Also, make sure that the collar is not too tight, and if your dog is still growing, check the collar every week to make sure the pet has not outgrown it.

In addition to an identification tag, you may wish to consider a form of permanent marking to ensure that your dog can be identified if its tags are accidentally or intentionally removed. Permanent marking includes a tattoo or a subcutaneous implant. If your dog is lost or stolen, these permanent markings will enable you to positively identify the pet as belonging to you, and a permanent marking should alert anyone who comes into contact with the pet that it is not an unwanted stray.

Dogs that spend most of their time outside and unsupervised or are permitted to roam have more exposure than confined dogs to poisons and risk a multitude of traumas, including injury from cars, guns, other animals and even people. In addition, dogs that are permitted to roam can pose a threat to people and other people's pets.

Unconfined dogs also have a higher risk of getting infections because of their increased exposure to disease. Infections like canine distemper, parainfluenza, leptospirosis, hepatitis, parvovirus, coronavirus, bordetella and rabies virus can be fatal. Parasitic infections can also cause serious disease.

When your dog is in your home, it is advisable to keep all windows at least partially closed to prevent your pet from accidentally or intentionally using a window as a door. Note that screens in windows may not be enough of a barrier to prevent your dog from falling or jumping through a window.

Outdoor precautions include providing the dog with fresh food and water. (Note that water may freeze quickly in the winter months.) In the cool months, the dog should have good shelter away from drafts and dampness. The shelter should be just big enough for the dog to lie down and to stand. Too much height, depth and length does not promote heat conservation. The shelter should contain clean, dry bedding, ideally straw. Wet or soiled bedding needs to be replaced immediately. When the temperature falls below freezing, your pet should be moved inside or provided with an alternative heat source like a heat lamp. Your dog's paws should be kept clean of ice, salt and mud. Because trapping is a cool weather sport, in the winter months it is especially important that your dog not be permitted to roam in any area where trapping may occur. Wooded areas, especially near creek beds, are common places for leg-hold traps to be set.

In the summer months, it is particularly important that if your dog is outdoors it has access to plenty of fresh water. If your dog sometimes tips over its water bowl, partially bury the bowl in the ground. Also, make sure your pet has adequate shade from summer mid-day heat. If your dog spends time in a shed or garage, good ventilation is essential. These special precautions during the summer months will help prevent potentially deadly heat stroke.

Because dogs have a tendency to eat grass, it is important to keep your dog indoors if your lawn has been chemically treated recently with pesticides or fertilizers. Lawn chemicals can poison a dog, or they may cause chemical burns to the pet's feet. Also, if you have recently sprayed insecticides inside your home, keep your dog out of the rooms that have been sprayed until the chemicals dissipate.

Even indoors, dogs are not without risk. Modifying their environment can help decrease the likelihood of emergencies. Dog-proof your home by removing potential hazards. Make sure electrical and other cords are not dangling in a manner that will entice your dog to chew on them. Electrical cords can cause severe burns or death if

13

your dog chews through the protective insulation, and any type of cord (e.g., telephone, drapery, etc.) poses a danger of strangulation. Also, keep your dog's toenails well-trimmed to prevent them from catching on carpets and furniture.

Make sure that any toy you give to your dog is constructed so that your dog cannot eat portions that may be nondigestible. If portions are missing, remove and replace the toy. No toys should have any strings dangling because ingested string can cut through a dog's digestive tract. All toys should be large enough and strong enough that neither the whole toy nor any part of it can be swallowed. Socks, hose and shoes with laces are also choking hazards and should be kept out of your dog's reach.

Dogs have a keen sense of smell, and ordinary household items can become hazards if they contain food smells. For example, a steel wool pad that you have used to scrub a pan after cooking bacon or some other meat can become a deadly enticement for your pet. Dogs will sometimes eat knives, forks and other utensils used to prepare foods. Even flavored dental floss is appetizing to some dogs, and dental floss may cause fatal bowel injuries if swallowed. Aluminum foil or any other wrap that has been used on any food product that might be appealing to your dog should be discarded in a manner that prevents your dog from having access to it. You should note that metal products like steel wool pads and aluminum foil are particularly destructive to a dog's digestive system. Similarly, Christmas-tree tinsel is extremely destructive to a dog's stomach and bowels, and you should never decorate a Christmas tree with tinsel if your dog has any chance of getting to the tree.

Toxic indoor plants should be identified and removed or kept out of reach. (See Part 5 - Poisonous Plants.) If your dog is permitted outside, to the extent possible you should attempt to limit its access to potentially harmful plants.

Never use a flea product on puppies if it is labeled for adult dogs only. Flea dips for adult dogs can be especially dangerous for puppies. Also, flea products for dogs can become toxic when not used properly. Always read and follow product labels carefully.

Never feed your dog chocolate, table scraps or bones. Chocolate is poisonous to dogs because it contains theobromine, which they cannot metabolize. In general, table scraps can predispose the dog to pancreatitis and other digestive upsets, and milk can be a major cause of diarrhea. Bones cannot be digested and can pierce the digestive-tract lining, possibly causing fatal peritonitis (inflammation within the abdomen). As a preventive measure, keep all people food away from your dog, and keep trash containers secured.

People medications are often poisonous to dogs, especially acetaminophen (Tylenol®) and ibuprofen, which are potentially lethal for canines. (See pages 54 and 105.) Never administer medications of any type without specific instructions from your veterinarian.

During transportation, do not allow your dog to ride on your lap, stand on the back window ledge or engage in any behavior that might detract from your attention to your driving or put the pet at additional risk in the event of an accident. Do not permit your dog to put its entire head out of the window; the wind from the moving car blows debris that can injure a dog's eyes. Also, never transport a dog in the back of an open pickup truck.

Finally, make sure your dog is up-to-date on its vaccinations. In addition to vaccinations, there are preventive medications that your dog may need. For example, heartworm disease, which is spread by mosquitoes, can be prevented by monthly medications. The appendix section on Preventive Health Care lists the vaccinations and medications that your dog should receive as well as a timetable for vaccinations and boosters and medications. You should note that many dog diseases that are easily preventable with a vaccine are often fatal, including rabies, which can be transmitted to people.

The reasonable precautions discussed above and outlined below should decrease the risk of an emergency and may save your dog's life.

I. Accident-Proofing your Home

A. Keep telephone cords, drapery cords and electrical cords out of reach.

B. Make sure that any dog toys are sufficiently large and indestructible that they do not pose a risk of choking. Also, make sure that they do not contain any string or yarn.

C. Make sure that your dog does not have access to socks, hose or shoes/shoelaces.

D. Do not decorate a Christmas tree with tinsel.

E. Keep all utensils, foils, wraps, scrub pads, etc. that may contain food smells out of reach of your dog.

F. Never give your dog human medications of any kind without specific instructions from a veterinarian. Acetaminophen

15

(Tylenol®) and ibuprofen can be fatal to your dog. Keep all medications out of your dog's reach.

G. Identify and remove toxic plants and flowers. (Refer to the Poisonous Plants chapter in this book.)

H. Keep your dog off of lawns that have been recently treated with pesticides or fertilizers.

I. Keep your dog out of rooms where you have recently sprayed indoor insecticides.

J. Never use snail bait, rat poison or poisonous ant traps.

K. Never use continual-release toilet disinfectants.

L. Keep windows above the ground floor at least partially closed.

M. Provide good ventilation during hot summer months.

N. Keep all trash containers covered, and keep any and all table scraps, especially bones, away from your dog.

II. Prevention for Outside the Home

A. Provide your dog with an identification tag.

B. Properly dispose of antifreeze.

C. Never use snail bait or rat poison.

D. When your dog is outside unsupervised, keep the pet in a secured area (i.e., secured with a fence or an invisible fence) or keep the dog tied.

E. Honk your car horn before pulling out of the driveway.

F. Identify and remove toxic plants and flowers. (Refer to the Poisonous Plants chapter in this book.)

G. In the winter, provide fresh water, and change it before it freezes.

H. In cool months, provide dry, draft-free shelter. The shelter should be just big enough for the dog to lie down and to stand; too much height, depth and length does not promote heat conservation and will not serve well as a shelter. Put bedding (i.e., clean, dry straw) in the shelter.

I. During hot summer months, provide well-ventilated shelter and extra drinking water.

III. Preventive Medicine

A. Keep vaccinations and physical exams up-to-date.

B. Get an annual heartworm test and heartworm preventive medicine.
C. Follow flea-product instructions carefully.
D. Never give any medication without a veterinarian's advice.
E. Never give your dog any people medications like acetaminophen (Tylenol®) or ibuprofen – these substances can be deadly.
F. Spay or neuter your dog.

IV. Additional Measures
A. Never leave a dog alone for an extended period of time.
B. Never leave a dog alone in a hot car with the windows up.
C. Keep hair coat free of mats (to prevent skin sores).
D. Keep paws free of ice, mud and salt; wash and dry the paws.
E. Never call your dog to come if the dog has to cross a road in front of cars. Instead, cross the street yourself, and then bring the dog to the other side with you.

V. Preventive Nutrition
A. Never feed dogs cat food. Cat food lacks the balance of nutrients essential for healthy dogs. Also, it may cause diarrhea, or the high fat content may promote obesity.
B. Never feed dogs milk. Milk can cause digestive problems like diarrhea.
C. Do not supplement diets without a veterinarian's advice. Wrong supplementation can cause urinary tract problems, metabolic problems and even mineralization of the kidneys.
D. Never feed a dog raw fish. Raw fish causes a thiamine deficiency which may result in loss of appetite, a hunched and painful stance and possibly convulsions. Even if it is cooked, never feed a dog a diet of fish exclusively.
E. Never feed a dog foods that contain rancid fats or excess polyunsaturated fats because they can cause a vitamin E deficiency leading to a variety of muscle diseases.
F. Never feed your dog table scraps, bones or chocolates.
G. Never oversupplement your dog's diet with vitamin D or fish liver oil. Excess can cause bone disease as well as digestive upset.

THE FIRST-AID KIT

The most important feature of a first-aid kit is accessibility. The kit must be readily available when an emergency occurs. Therefore, it is important to keep the kit in a location that is obvious (e.g., beside the dog food) and in a location that provides easy access, such as an unlocked drawer or cupboard. The items in a kit should be kept within a container that is easily transported, in case you need to bring the kit to the dog. Finally, the kit should be in a closed container that will keep its contents clean and dry. A fishing tackle or utility box would be a good choice.

Once you have selected a suitable container for the kit, it is time to stock it with the items you will most likely need in an emergency. First, stock your kit with three large plastic garbage bags to protect car upholstery and household furnishings from blood, urine and feces. Then include 2 rolls of 3" gauze bandage and 12 gauze sponges 3"x3" for wound care. Obtain adhesive tape of the non-stick type; it will provide more comfort to your dog than ordinary tape that sticks to hair. Next, add scissors and toenail trimmers, several paper towels (for cleaning up messes), antibiotic ointment, saline solution (the kind people use for contact-lens cleaning), Benedryl® or diphenhydramine elixir (12.5 mg/ml liquid), tweezers, an eyedropper (for use in force-feeding liquid medications), a rectal thermometer, nonstick bandages, alcohol and hydrogen peroxide. Also include a dog muzzle, preferably the nylon variety as opposed to a leather one. A nylon muzzle is more comfortable for your pet and can be laundered easily. In a pinch you can construct a muzzle from gauze or a gentleman's necktie (see page 45 in the First-Aid Techniques section of this book), but a homemade muzzle will be more difficult to use on your dog and may not work as well.

Other items that are useful but will not fit into your first-aid container should be kept in close proximity to the kit. Make sure you have two 2-liter soda bottles that you can fill with warm water in an emergency to help keep your dog from getting chilled. Also have access to clean bath towels and a blanket to aid in transportation and restraint and to provide warmth. Finally, if you have a small dog, get a pet carrier so that you can safely transport your pet in an emergency. If you have a small dog and are unable to obtain a pet carrier, make sure you have a ventilated box that is the appropriate size and is suitably durable to serve as a substitute.

18

To ensure you have easy access to professional help, make a list of telephone numbers of the pet's daytime veterinarian, a reserve day-time veterinarian, two night-time veterinary emergency numbers, the local poison control hotline, and the National Animal Poison Control Center. (The National Animal Poison Control Center provides assistance for a fee - $20 for 5 minutes at the time of this printing: 1-900-680-0000.) Put one copy of the list in your first-aid kit and another near the telephone.

I. First-Aid Box

A. Obtain a box that is
    (1) Transportable (shoe-box size, preferably with a handle)
    (2) Durable and water-resistant (like a fishing tackle box)
    (3) Non-locking (to provide easy access).
B. Label the outside of the box "DOG FIRST AID".
C. Store the first-aid box in plain view.

II. First-Aid Provisions (to put into First-Aid Box)

A. 2 rolls of 3" gauze bandage
B. 12 gauze sponges 3"x 3"
C. Nonstick adhesive tape
D. Nonstick bandages
E. Antibiotic ointment (e.g., Polysporin®) – small tube
F. Water-soluble lubricating jelly (e.g., K-Y™ Brand)
G. Saline solution – 8 ounces (same as used for contact-lens care)
H. Hydrogen peroxide – 8 ounces
I. Alcohol
J. Eyedropper or dosage syringe
K. Tweezers
L. Scissors
M. Nail trimmers
N. Rectal thermometer
O. Muzzle – preferably nylon
P. Benedryl® or diphenhydramine elixir (12.5 mg/ml liquid)
Q. Paper towels – to clean up any mess

R. 3 large garbage bags

S. Emergency information (see below)

III. Emergency Information

A. Emergency telephone numbers:

    (1) Poison control _____

    (2) Veterinarians _____

    _____

    (3) After-hours veterinarians _____

    _____

    (4) Fire department _____

B. A copy of this book

C. A copy of the First-Aid Provisions List

D. A plant identification book

IV. Additional First-Aid Items

A. Towels – for use in restraining your dog

B. Blanket – to keep your dog warm and comfortable

C. Pet carrier – for transport if you have a dog

D. A plywood board cut to the appropriate size for your dog and for your car – to carry your injured dog safely to the car

E. Two 2-liter soda bottles – for use as hot-water bottles

HOW TO APPROACH AN EMERGENCY

When an emergency occurs, the first step is to decide whether to become directly involved. Evaluate the risk to you, the dog and others. Be conscious of the surroundings. For example, if you are driving and you see an injured dog at the side of the highway, first consider whether there is a safe place to stop, and then consider whether the situation could get worse if the dog runs when you try to approach it. If the overall risk is too great, call a professional (i.e., an animal shelter, the humane society or a veterinarian).

Pet emergencies are stressful, and your anxiety can interfere with your common sense. It is important to stay as calm as possible during an emergency in order to give your dog the best care. If you become too emotional, it may be advisable to have a family member or friend help provide care. Remember that your pet is totally dependent upon you during an emergency.

One of the most important actions you can take prior to an emergency is to make arrangements to have access to veterinary care 24 hours a day. This may take some planning, especially if you live in a rural area. Most large cities have pet emergency-care centers. Even though the pet may have a regular veterinarian, it is a good idea to have at least one other doctor available as a backup during the day. Also, make arrangements to have two night-time veterinarians available. In selecting your emergency veterinary numbers, it is important for you to consider not only the skills of the veterinarians but also their locations. The closer the doctor's office, the better the pet's chances if a problem occurs in which time is a factor. The veterinarians' telephone numbers should be listed near the phone as well as in your first-aid kit.

Make sure any pet sitter understands the emergency instructions. The pet sitter should know whom to contact in case of an emergency. The dog's doctor should also be notified of treatment preferences in the event of an emergency when the owner is unavailable; otherwise the veterinarian will likely provide only basic care until given permission to proceed with additional treatments.

Regardless of the emergency, there are some basic steps you can take to help your dog. The following information should enable you to take appropriate action in a variety of emergency situations.

21

I. Basic Steps in Emergency Care

A. Stay calm. Focus on the dog's needs. Use common sense during the crisis. If you are unable to deal with the situation, then delegate the emergency care to someone else.

B. Observe the urgency. Does the emergency appear to be mild, moderate, or severe? Evaluate whether the situation is getting better, staying the same, or getting worse.

C. Seek assistance:

    (1) Call the dog's doctor.

    (2) If the emergency occurs outside of regular veterinary hours, call for after-hour help.

    (3) If you suspect poisoning and cannot reach a veterinarian, call your local poison control hotline or the National Animal Poison Control Center. (The National Animal Poison Control Center provides assistance for a fee – $20 for 5 minutes at the time of this printing: 1-900-680-0000.)

    (4) If no professional help is available, proceed to Step II.

II. First-Aid Instructions

A. Identify the problem or symptom; then refer to the alphabetically-arranged emergency section or to the index of this book.

B. If the problem cannot be identified, follow these steps:

    (1) Confine the dog.

    (2) Keep the dog quiet and warm.

    (3) Note any and all symptoms.

    (4) Observe whether the condition is getting better, staying the same or getting worse.

    (5) Refer to the Emergency Worksheet on page 286 for additional help.

C. Contact a veterinarian as soon as possible.

RESTRAINT

Hurt or sick pets may react unpredictably; often instinctual behavior overrides normal disposition. This is important to remember when your pet needs special handling or treatment during an emergency. Dogs usually respond to illness in one of three ways: some will not show behavioral changes and will respond to handling in their normal manner; others may become listless or depressed, in which case they tend to be relatively easy to handle; and others may become anxious or aggressive, an instinctive reaction often associated with pain and fear. This instinctive reaction can make handling and treatment very difficult. When an anxious dog struggles, it poses a risk of injury to the caretaker; a scared dog will often bite.

Struggling dogs also pose a risk of further injuring themselves. In cases where the dog is frightened, is in obvious pain or is behaving aggressively, your approach and handling techniques are important. Approach an anxious or aggressive dog slowly and calmly, talking quietly to the pet. Repeat "good dog", "good girl" or "good boy". If the dog tries to flee and will not obey your commands, your first step is to decide whether to intervene. There is often a risk to both the dog and you in this situation. In addition, a dog that is not vaccinated may carry rabies, a disease that can be fatal to people. If you make the decision not to intervene, you may wish to employ the help of a professional such as a house-call veterinarian or a humane-society volunteer. These professionals are proficient at dealing with hard-to-handle dogs.

Always approach a dog from behind to avoid being bitten. Once the dog is in hand, the pet can be lifted or positioned for further care or examination. See illustration on page 25. If the dog is fighting, this method of restraint may cause risk of injury, and you should consider using a large towel or blanket instead of your hands (i.e., place the towel or blanket over the pet, and gather the pet in the towel/blanket to complete the restraint). Slowly approach the pet (from behind, if possible) and place the towel or blanket over the dog. If a fracture, neck or back injury is suspected, take care to avoid excessive movement of the dog. Movement can be minimized by sliding the pet onto a small board or directly into a pet carrier.

If you follow the rules for several basic restraint techniques, the stress during an emergency will be decreased for the pet and for you.

I. Behavioral Changes Affecting Restraint of the Sick, Hurt Dog

A. Listless or depressed dogs may be easier to handle.

B. Hurt or sick dogs may become anxious or aggressive and be more difficult to handle. They may bite.

C. Some dogs may not show behavioral changes and may be predictable to handle.

II. Approaching an Injured Dog

A. Talk to the dog calmly and quietly.

B. Move toward the dog slowly.

C. Do not chase the dog.

III. Restraining the Injured Dog

A. Obtain a towel (for a small dog) or blanket (for a large dog) and a muzzle.

B. Approach from behind to help prevent getting bitten.

C. If the dog is trying to bite, use a muzzle, unless the dog is having trouble breathing or has been vomiting. Never muzzle a pet that is having breathing difficulty or is nauseated! Do not use a muzzle if your dog has a flat face (e.g., a pug, boxer, English bulldog, etc.). See pages 45-47.
Caution: dogs can bite through virtually any gloves, and even a friendly dog may bite when it is injured!

D. Place the towel or blanket over the dog.

E. Gather the dog in the towel or blanket to complete the restraint.

F. To carry or transport the dog, see Transportation, pages 26-29.

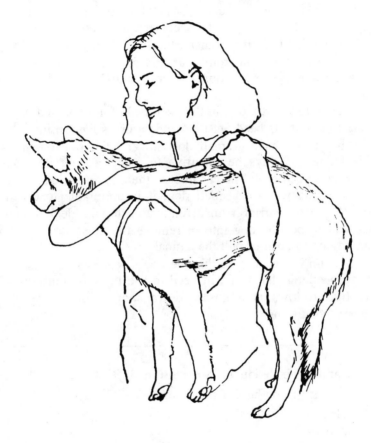

TRANSPORTATION

Transporting an injured or sick dog can sometimes be as stressful and hazardous to the dog as the emergency itself. A dog that normally enjoys riding in a car may not like being in the car under emergency conditions. It may be necessary, therefore, to have the dog properly restrained during transportation. See pages 23-25. In addition to distracting you from your driving, an unrestricted injured dog is at greater risk of additional injury from losing its balance and falling.

Never transport a dog in the open bed of a truck, and never let your dog ride with its head out the window or its feet on the window edge. And if you have a small dog, never let it ride on the back window ledge. Always be sensitive to whether your dog is in a relatively safe position in the car in case there is an accident or other driving emergency. For a small dog, it is preferable to use a pet carrier. A plastic carrier with a removable top is ideal because it enables you to put the dog into or remove the dog from the carrier without having to push or pull the animal.

It is important to note that the dog's condition will dictate the specific procedures that you will need to use for safe transport. The outline that follows is a guide to transport under a variety of emergency conditions.

I.   Equipment Needed in Transportation

A.   Pet carrier (if you have a small dog)

B.   Towels

C.   Blanket

D.   2-liter soda bottle filled with warm water

E.   Muzzle

F.   Collar and leash

G.   Car safety belt for dogs (optional)

H.   Plywood board cut to fit your dog and your car

II.   Carrying an Injured Dog

A.   Even a friendly dog may bite when it is in pain. Therefore, apply a muzzle if the dog is not having difficulty breathing and has not been vomiting. Do not use a muzzle if your dog has a flat face (e.g., a pug, boxer, English bulldog, etc.). See pages 45-47.

B. **For a small dog:**
   (1) Obtain a pet carrier that has a removable top. If a pet carrier is not available, use a corrugated cardboard box of an appropriate size. A carrier or box that opens at the top rather than the side is preferable because the dog can be put in and taken out without pushing or pulling the pet.
   (2) Slide your hands under the dog to lift the pet. Take care to support the dog's entire body as you lift and place the dog into the carrier.
   (3) Place towels around the dog to keep the pet from sliding in the pet carrier.

C. **For a medium-size or large dog:**
   (1) For spinal cord injuries, the risk of additional injury from moving the dog is substantial. The ideal carrying method is to slide the dog onto a plywood board and then secure the pet with a blanket. You will need someone to assist you in carrying the board. Make sure the board will fit in the vehicle you plan to use for transport.
   (2) For emergencies other than spinal cord injuries, you may still need to use a board (as detailed immediately above) if the dog is too large for you to carry by yourself. If the dog is not too large for you to carry by yourself, place one arm under the dog's stomach (below the ribs) and the other hand under the dog's neck (with the dog's neck in the corner of your elbow). See the illustration on page 25. When lifting the dog, bend your knees and lift with equal pressure on both arms.

III. Transporting a Dog in Stable Condition

A. For your own driving safety:
   (1) The dog should ride in the seat next to the driver or in the

back, and never in the driver's lap or near the pedals.

    (2) Restrain and secure the pet with a leash or a special dog safety belt, or, for a small dog, you may have a helper hold the pet.

B. For your dog's safety:

    (1) Never allow the pet to ride with its head outside the window or with its paws on the window's edge.

    (2) Never allow a small dog to ride on the back window ledge.

    (3) Never drive with your dog in the open bed of a truck.

IV. Transporting a Dog in Shock

A. If the dog is in pain, you may wish to use a muzzle. However, use a muzzle only if the dog is not having difficulty breathing and has not been vomiting. If at any time the dog has difficulty breathing, remove the muzzle. Also, do not use a muzzle if your dog has a flat face (e.g., a pug, boxer, English bulldog, etc.).

B. Lay the dog on the seat of the car. Pack blankets around the dog to keep the pet warm. If you are concerned that the dog may slide off of the seat onto the floor, pack the floor area with a pillow or blankets. Place one or two 2-liter soda bottles filled with warm water (not hot water) against the dog. See illustrations on pages 125-126.

V. Transporting a Dog with Fractures or Back Injuries

A. Plan the transport carefully to minimize movement of the dog.

B. Because fractures are painful, you may wish to use a muzzle to prevent being bitten when you move your dog. However, use a muzzle only if the dog is not having difficulty breathing and has not been vomiting. If at any time the dog has difficulty breathing, remove the muzzle. Also, do not use a muzzle if your dog has a flat face (e.g., a pug, boxer, English bulldog, etc.)

C. **For a small dog:**

    (1) Obtain a pet carrier that has a removable top. If a pet carrier is not available, use a corrugated cardboard box of an appropriate size. A carrier or box that opens at the top rather than the side is preferable because the dog can be put

in and taken out without pushing or pulling the pet.

(2) Slide your hands under the dog to lift the pet. Take care to support the dog's entire body as you lift. Place the dog into the carrier with its injured side up, if possible.

(3) Place towels around the dog to keep the pet from sliding in the pet carrier. Place a 2-liter soda bottle filled with warm water (not hot water) against the dog. See illustration on page 125.

D. **For a medium-size or large dog:**

(1) Obtain a plywood board that will fit easily into your car to use as a stretcher. Slide the dog onto the board taking care to move the pet as little as possible. If a board is not available, you may use a blanket or towel as a stretcher instead, but the board is highly preferable because it will result in less movement of the pet and therefore less chance of aggravating the injury.

(2) Ideally, place the plywood board with the dog on it into your vehicle. If the board will not fit, slide the dog off of the board and onto the seat with as little movement of the pet as possible. If you have used a blanket or towel rather than a board, keep the blanket or towel under the dog when you put the pet into the car.

(3) Pack blankets around the dog to keep the pet warm. If you are concerned that the dog may slide off of the seat onto the floor, pack the floor area with a pillow or blankets. Place one or two 2-liter soda bottles filled with warm water (not hot water) against the dog. See illustrations on pages 125-126.

SPECIAL CONSIDERATIONS

"Special considerations" refers to conditions that may complicate emergency treatment. In particular, this chapter will address the special needs of puppies, older dogs and dogs with preexisting diseases or medical conditions. Because each dog has unique characteristics, you should consult your veterinarian regarding any special treatment or special considerations in the day-to-day care of your pet as well as in emergency situations.

Because of the vast number of special considerations and the unique characteristics of each dog, this chapter can only begin to address the particular needs of your pet. If you suspect that your dog has special needs, find out now before an emergency develops so that you can administer the best possible care for your pet.

I. Puppies

A. Because of a puppy's small body size, it has little reserve to support itself during an illness.

B. Puppies have immature immune systems that are inadequate for fighting infections after the puppies are weaned from their mothers. Make sure your puppy gets timely vaccinations.

C. Because of a puppy's curiosity, it is prone to finding trouble that can result in injury.

II. Older Dogs

A. Older dogs require special care because their organs/internal functions may be diseased or show aging changes making them more sensitive to disease processes.

B. Make sure older dogs have easy access to food and water.

C. Some older dogs are prone to becoming underweight; therefore, they have less body reserve than fit dogs.

D. Other older dogs are overweight, which can predispose them to diseases and slow their recoveries.

E. Dogs over 7-8 years of age should have annual blood tests to screen for early diseases of the internal organs, diabetes and anemias. X-rays and an EKG may be warranted to identify early heart disease.

III. Preexisting Diseases

A. Obesity may predispose a dog to early heart, liver and kidney disease. It may also cause problems with early arthritis.

B. Metabolic disease problems (e.g., thyroid disorders, diabetes) can complicate recoveries if the diseases are not properly diagnosed and treated.

C. Heartworm disease may debilitate a dog and lead to chronic fatigue and heart and liver failure. The dog's weakened condition may make any emergency more urgent and may slow any recovery from illness or injury.

D. Other parasitic diseases (i.e., worms and protozoa) can weaken your dog and make any emergency even more critical.

IV. Body Shape and Size

A. Dogs with flat faces (e.g., pug, boxer, English bulldog, etc.) may have difficulty breathing when they are under stress and may overheat quickly. Therefore, do not muzzle a dog that has a flat face.

B. Some dogs have underdeveloped or small nostrils (e.g., pugs, Pekinese, Lhaso apso, Shih Tzu). Never use a muzzle on these dogs.

C. Deep-chested dogs (e.g., Irish setters, Great Danes, German shepherds, etc.) may be predisposed to twisted stomachs. See pages 69-70.

D. Obesity may predispose a dog to early heart, liver and kidney disease. It may also cause problems with early arthritis.

31

PART 2

FIRST-AID TECHNIQUES

INTRODUCTION TO TECHNIQUES

There are many techniques that you should practice and learn now so that you will know them in the event of an emergency. Repetition and mental preparation will enable you to cope with the stress of an emergency in a more organized manner and will enable you to perform necessary techniques more efficiently.

The eight techniques described in this chapter are presented in logical order: external, internal and other. Bleeding control, wound care and wrapping a wound comprise the external techniques. These three techniques are essential elements of emergency treatment for lacerations, abrasions, bite wounds and a variety of other traumas. Monitoring vital signs (i.e., temperature, pulse and respiration), inducing vomiting and performing cardiopulmonary resuscitation are the three techniques that involve a dog's internal systems. Monitoring vital signs serves in both diagnosis of a problem as well as in the evaluation of severity and change in condition. Inducing vomiting is a procedure that applies to a multitude of situations involving poisoning; it is, in many circumstances, a life-saving technique. Cardiopulmonary resuscitation (CPR) is a technique used in the most critical situations when your dog has stopped breathing and has no pulse. When CPR is necessary, there is no time to find a veterinarian, which means that your ability to perform the technique will determine whether your dog has a chance of surviving.

The two remaining techniques involve construction and use of simple restraining devices: the muzzle and the Elizabethan collar. The muzzle is used primarily to facilitate safe handling of the pet (i.e., to prevent the dog from biting you or someone else), whereas the Elizabethan collar is used to keep the pet from licking or biting itself. Both devices are used in a variety of situations, and it is therefore important that you either purchase a commercial variety of each or else use the instructions in this book to construct home-made versions.

BLEEDING CONTROL

Often an emergency involves some type of hemorrhage (i.e., bleeding). The bleeding may be mild, moderate, or severe. Severe hemorrhage may involve the severing of an artery, injury to a large muscle mass, a fracture of a bone, toxicity due to rat poisoning, or internal trauma to an organ. If the blood pools quickly or pumps in spurts, you can assume it is serious. Immediate action is required to prevent shock.

I. **First-Aid Materials**

A. Clean towel

B. Gauze sponges

C. Nonstick adhesive tape

D. Nonstick bandages

E. Gauze wrap

II. **Technique Instructions**

A. Locate the source of bleeding.

B. Using a clean towel or gauze sponges, apply firm direct pressure to the wound for 5-10 minutes.

C. Note how fast the blood pools or if it spurts. Make an observation of the amount of blood loss.

D. A wrap may be applied to the area if hemorrhage has slowed. (See page 37 on Wrapping a Wound.) DO NOT attempt to clean the wound or apply antibiotic ointment because the clot may be disrupted and severe hemorrhage may resume.

III. **Emergency Situations Where the Technique Applies**

A. Open fractures

B. Bite wounds

C. Abrasions

D. Lacerations

E. Other trauma, such as gunshot wounds

WOUND CARE

Proper cleansing of wounds can facilitate healing and help prevent infection. Many minor wounds can be treated at home, but they should be checked by a veterinarian who may recommend antibiotics.

I. First-Aid Materials

A. Saline solution (i.e., contact-lens saline solution)

B. Mild antibacterial soap

C. Water-soluble lubricating jelly (e.g., K-Y™ Brand)

D. Clippers or scissors

E. Antibiotic ointment (e.g., Polysporin®)

II. Technique Instructions

A. Apply water-soluble lubricating jelly to the wound to protect it from the pet's hair and to protect it from further contamination.

B. Using clippers or carefully using scissors, trim the dog's hair from around the wound.

C. Using water or saline solution, rinse the lubricating jelly from the wound.

D. If the wound is visibly soiled, rinse it with water until all debris is removed. Be careful not to rinse surrounding debris into the wound.

E. Gently scrub the area using antibacterial soap and water. Rinse well with water, then with saline solution if available.

F. Apply antibiotic ointment. If necessary to keep the wound clean, apply a wrap. (See Wrapping a Wound on page 37.)

III. Emergencies Situations Where the Technique Applies

A. Burns

B. Abrasions

C. Lacerations

D. Bite wounds

E. Other trauma

WRAPPING A WOUND

Wraps should be applied to areas where abrasions or lacerations are present to keep them clean and to prevent the dog from causing further trauma by licking a wound. In many situations where a wrap is needed, an Elizabethan collar may also be necessary. See page 48.

I. **First-Aid Materials**
A. Antibiotic ointment (e.g., Polysporin®)
B. Saline solution
C. Nonstick adhesive tape
D. Nonstick bandages
E. Gauze wrap

II. **Technique Instructions**
A. Treat the injury according to the specific instructions provided elsewhere in this book (e.g., Wound Care on page 36).
B. Apply antibiotic ointment over wound.
C. Press nonstick bandage to wound.
D. Secure nonstick bandage to wound by wrapping gauze around the leg or body. The gauze should be pulled snug but not tight. The wrap tightness should not restrict circulation or the dog's breathing.
E. Secure the gauze by applying adhesive tape to the wrap.
F. Monitor the pet for any evidence of swelling to the limb below the wrap. If swelling occurs, then the wrap is too tight and should be removed immediately. If the dog's breathing is hindered, also remove the wrap.

III. **Emergency Situations Where the Technique Applies**
A. Abrasions
B. Lacerations
C. Burns
D. Other skin irritations
E. Compound/open fractures

MONITORING VITAL SIGNS (TEMPERATURE, PULSE AND RESPIRATIONS)

Monitoring vital signs gives the veterinarian and pet owner a basis for evaluating the pet's progress during an illness. The techniques for obtaining pulse and respirations are noninvasive, but unfortunately taking the pet's temperature is a procedure that not every dog will tolerate and not every caretaker may feel comfortable performing. The decision to obtain a temperature from a pet should be based on the pet's disposition and the owner's willingness to participate.

I.   **First-Aid Materials**

A.   Rectal thermometer

B.   Water-soluble lubricating jelly (e.g., K-Y™ Brand) or petroleum jelly

C.   Watch or clock with second hand

II. **Technique Instructions**

A.   Taking the temperature:

(1) Lubricate a rectal thermometer with water-soluble lubricating jelly or petroleum jelly. Insert the thermometer gently into the dog's rectum approximately 1 inch.

(2) Wait 2 minutes, and then remove and read the thermometer.

(3) Normal temperature is between 101 and 103 degrees Fahrenheit.

B.   Taking the pulse:

(1) Lay your hand just behind the dog's shoulder blade on either side of its chest and feel for the heart beat (as illustrated on page 44), or

(2) Place your hand in the groin area of the dog's abdomen and

feel for the femoral pulse.

    (3) Count the beats per minute (e.g., count for 15 seconds and multiply by 4).

    (4) Normal pulse at rest should range from approximately 100 to 130 beats per minute. If the dog has been recently active or is excited, its pulse may be significantly higher.

C.   Taking respirations:

    (1) If the dog is lying quietly, watch the chest rise and fall.

    (2) Count the number of breaths the dog takes in a minute.

    (3) Normal resting respiratory rate is approximately 20 to 24 breaths per minute.

III. Emergency Situations Where the Technique Applies

A.   Virtually all conditions

INDUCING VOMITING

When a dog ingests a poisonous substance, time is critical, and your ability to induce your dog to vomit may save its life.

NOTE: Vomiting should NEVER be induced if a pet is unconscious or in a stupor. Also never induce vomiting if there is suspicion of ingestion of petroleum distillates, acids or alkalis (e.g., kerosene, gasoline, motor oil, various household cleaning supplies). As a general rule, follow the instructions on the product warning label regarding whether to induce vomiting. If in doubt, call a poison control center, but make sure you act quickly.

I. **First-Aid Materials**

A. Hydrogen peroxide

B. Eyedropper or dosage syringe

II. **Technique Instructions**

A. Induce vomiting only if the dog is conscious. Before proceeding, attempt to contact your veterinarian. If a veterinarian is not immediately available, then feed the dog 1 teaspoon of hydrogen peroxide (mixed with 1 teaspoon of milk if available). If the dog will not drink the mixture or if there is no milk available, then force-feed the dog the hydrogen peroxide using an eyedropper.

B. If vomiting does not occur within 10 minutes, repeat the procedure twice if needed.

C. Contact a veterinarian as soon as possible.

III. **Emergencies Situations Where the Technique Applies**

A. Most poisonings. (See note above.)

CARDIOPULMONARY RESUSCITATION

Just like in human medicine, cardiopulmonary resuscitation (CPR) for your dog can mean the difference between life and death. This technique may enable a critically-injured dog to survive until it is transported to a veterinary hospital.

CPR is used to revive a dog that is not breathing and has no heartbeat (e.g., from drowning or severe electrical shock). When CPR is needed, it must be performed immediately. Therefore, it is imperative that you be able to assess the need quickly and perform the technique effectively.

Unlike many other emergency techniques, cardiopulmonary resuscitation is performed without any special equipment or materials.

NOTE: CPR is a technique of last resort when the dog shows no signs of life. If there is any evidence that the dog is breathing, do not perform this technique.

I. **Technique Instructions**

A. Lay the dog on its side (and throughout these procedures keep the dog on its side).

B. Check for breathing by watching the dog's chest rise and fall.

C. **If the dog is breathing**, proceed no further. Do not use CPR.

D. **If the dog is not breathing,**

    (1) Establish an airway by removing any debris from the dog's mouth or by moving the tongue from the back of the throat. (See illustration page 42.) Check for breathing by watching the dog's chest rise and fall. If the dog is breathing, proceed no further, and do not use CPR.

    (2) Check for a pulse by placing a hand over the dog's chest just behind the shoulder blade (see illustration on page 44) to feel the heartbeat or by placing a hand in the groin area to feel the femoral pulse.

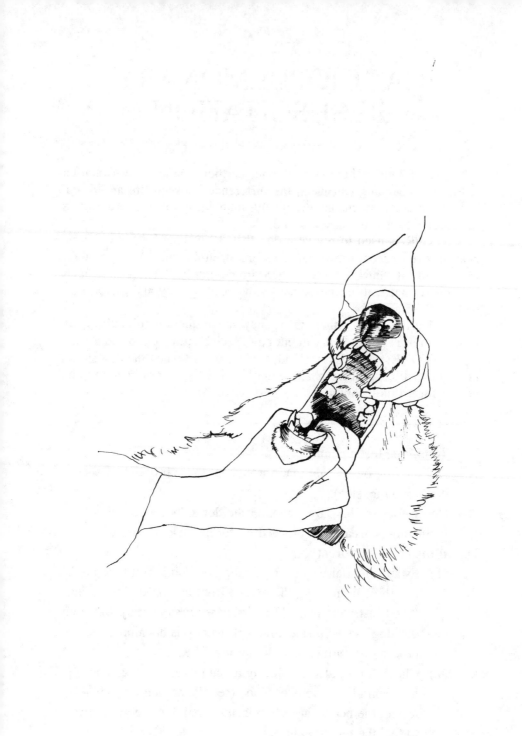

E. **If the dog still is not breathing,**

   (1) Cup your hand(s) over the dog's nose and mouth to form a seal. Deliver 1 breath into the pet every 2 seconds. If the seal is proper, you should observe the dog's chest rise and fall.

   (2) If after you have delivered 5 breaths the dog does not show signs of breathing on its own or signs of consciousness, and there is no heartbeat, then have a helper place a hand just behind the dog's shoulder blades (as illustrated on page 44), and apply gentle but firm compressions downward (compressing 1/2 to 1 inch for a small dog up to as much as 2 inches for a large dog) at a rate of 1 compression every 2 seconds. If a helper is not available, alternate delivering 2 breaths then 10 compressions. Do not do any compressions if there is a pulse, no matter how faint.

   (3) Check for a pulse and breathing every 2 minutes. If there is no pulse and breathing, continue for up to 10 minutes before giving up.

II. **Emergency Situations Where the Technique Applies**

A. Heart disease

B. Seizures

C. Trauma

D. Lung disease

E. Heat stroke

F. Shock

G. Poisonings

H. Any other circumstances that cause the heart to stop

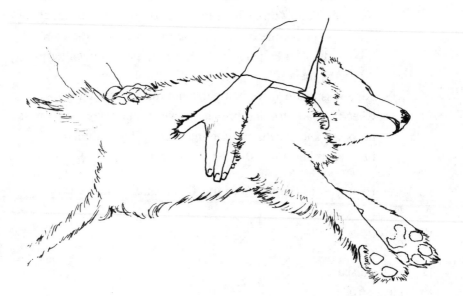

HOW TO MUZZLE A DOG

It may be necessary in certain cases to rely on a muzzle to help prevent a dog from biting when the dog is injured or extremely ill. A commercial muzzle is highly preferable to a homemade muzzle because it is easier to use and is often more effective. If a commercial muzzle is not available, however, a homemade muzzle is simple to construct.

NOTE: Never apply a muzzle if the dog is having difficulty breathing or is vomiting. Also, never apply a muzzle to a dog that has a flat face or small nostrils.

I.   First-Aid Materials

A.   A commercial muzzle, or

B.   Materials to make a homemade muzzle:
    (1)   1 strip of gauze (3 feet long for a little dog or up to 6 feet long for a big dog)
    (2)   Scissors

II.   Making a Homemade Muzzle

A.   Double the gauze strip and then tie a loose loop with the material. See the illustration on page 46.

B.   Approach the dog from the rear and slip this loop quickly over the dog's nose guiding it back toward the corners of the mouth. Make the loop snug, but do not pinch the dog.

C.   Then with the ends of the gauze strips, wrap the gauze around to the bottom of the dog's mouth, and then tie it behind the dog's ears. See the illustration on page 47.

III.   Using a Muzzle

A.   Approach the dog from behind and apply the muzzle quickly.

B.   With either a commercial or a homemade muzzle, it is helpful to have someone hold the dog's front feet down so the pet won't pull off the muzzle.

C. Be prepared to remove the muzzle promptly if the dog has difficulty breathing or if there is any indication that the dog might vomit.

IV. Emergency Situations Where the Technique Applies

A. Trauma

B. Any situation where the dog is difficult to handle

C. Never apply a muzzle if the dog is having difficulty breathing or is vomiting.

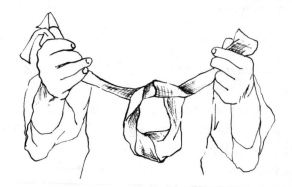

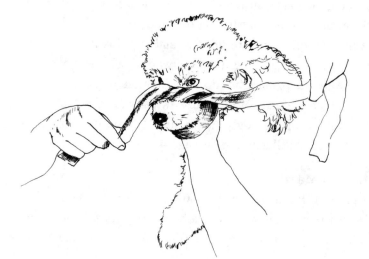

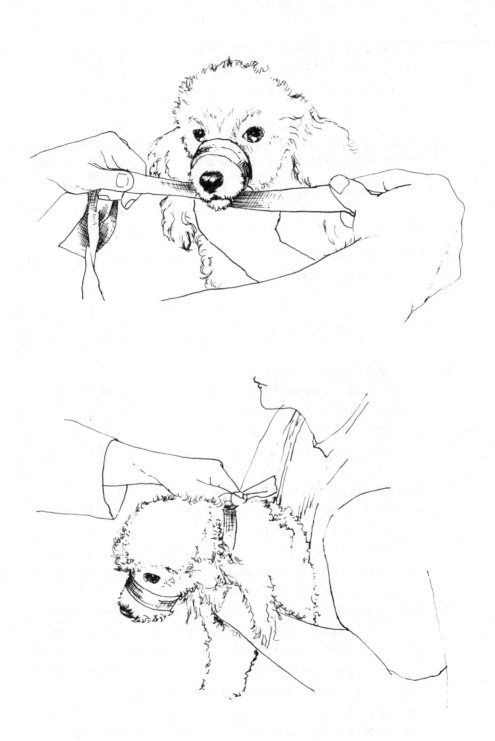

ELIZABETHAN COLLAR

An Elizabethan collar is a cone-shaped device that fits around the dog's neck. It is used to prevent a dog from instinctively licking or chewing an external injury. Because the dog's licking or chewing can cause additional damage and promote infection, the Elizabethan collar can help prevent serious complications.

I. **First-Aid Materials**

A. Medium-weight cardboard

B. Tape

C. Scissors

D. Or instead of the above items, a commercial Elizabethan collar

II. **Technique Instructions**

A. To construct a homemade Elizabethan collar, perform the following (as illustrated on page 50):

   (1) Draw a circle on the cardboard (8 inches in diameter for a small dog with a small nose, up to 20 inches in diameter for a large dog with a long nose).

   (2) Cut out this circle.

   (3) Cut a circular hole the size of the dog's neck out of the center of the larger circle.

   (4) Make one cut from the outside diameter to the inside hole.

   (5) Slip the cardboard cut-out over the pet's head and secure the edges with tape to form a cone-like shape.

B. Fasten the collar securely, but make sure that it does not impede the dog's breathing. It should be loose enough for you to slip two fingers under the collar. The collar should be long enough to keep the pet from licking and chewing. It may take the dog some time to get used to the collar while walking, eating, and drinking.

C. Make sure the dog will eat and drink while wearing its collar.

III. Emergency Situations Where the Technique Applies

A. Skin irritations
B. Protruding organs
C. Bite wounds
D. Traumas
E. Other problems where the dog may make an injury worse by licking or chewing

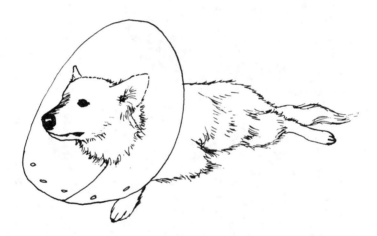

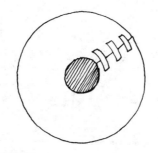

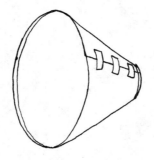

PART 3

—

HELP FOR THE PROBLEM

INTRODUCTORY
INFORMATION

Part 3 of this book is designed to provide a quick reference for treating many emergencies. Although this material does apply to a wide variety of emergencies, there are situations that may fall outside the scope of this book.

Part 3 of this book will enable you to find information in two ways: (1) by looking up the disease or condition, or (2) by looking up the primary symptom you observe. All information in both sections is in alphabetical order.

For simplicity, we use the term "symptom" to refer to both symptoms (things observed or experienced from the dog's point of view) and signs (things observed from the person's point of view). Note that for any given disease or condition, some or all of the symptoms listed may be present. Logically, the more symptoms you observe, the more likely you are to make a proper diagnosis. However, because there are many totally different diseases and conditions that have similar symptoms, it is important that you contact a veterinarian as soon as possible to ensure a proper diagnosis.

PROBLEM/CONDITION – ABRASIONS

I. **Symptoms (some or all may be present)**
A. Red skin
B. Missing hair
C. Painful area

II. **First-Aid Materials**
A. Contact-lens saline solution or water
B. Antibacterial soap
C. Clippers or scissors
D. Antibiotic ointment (e.g., Polysporin®)
E. Wrap material and/or Elizabethan collar

III. **First Aid**
A. Clip hair away from abrasion.
B. Cleanse the abrasion using soap and saline solution or water.
C. Apply antibiotic ointment to the abrasion.
D. If necessary, apply a wrap over the abrasion and/or use an Elizabethan collar to keep the dog from licking, scratching or chewing the area. See page 37 on Wrapping a Wound and page 48 on how to make an Elizabethan collar.
E. Seek veterinary help if the dog's discomfort persists.

PROBLEM/CONDITION – ACETAMINOPHEN (TYLENOL®) TOXICITY

Like many human drugs, Tylenol® is toxic to dogs. No medications of any kind should be given to a dog without instructions from a veterinarian. And because dogs are curious by nature, all drugs should be kept out of your dog's reach to prevent accidental ingestion.

I. **Symptoms (some or all may be present)**
A. Listlessness
B. Difficult breathing
C. Vomiting and/or diarrhea
D. Dark-colored urine

II. **First-Aid Materials**
A. Hydrogen peroxide
B. Eyedropper or dosage syringe

III. **First Aid**
A. If the dog is conscious, induce vomiting immediately by feeding the pet 1 teaspoon of hydrogen peroxide (mixed with 1 teaspoon milk if available). If the dog will not drink the mixture or if there is no milk available, then force-feed the dog the hydrogen peroxide using an eyedropper. If vomiting does not occur within 10 minutes, repeat the procedure up to two times.
B. Contact a veterinarian for further treatment regardless of whether you are successful at inducing your dog to vomit.

PROBLEM/CONDITION – ALLERGIES

Allergies in dogs can be caused by a number of irritants. In people, allergies often cause sneezing, runny eyes, and wheezing, whereas in dogs allergies usually cause itching and rashes.

Some skin irritations would not be considered life-threatening emergencies, but the degree of discomfort for the dog may be great. This section applies to both skin emergencies and minor skin irritations.

I. Symptoms (some or all may be present)

A. Red skin

B. Excess shedding

C. Missing hair

D. Painful area

E. Dog scratching itself

II. First-Aid Materials

A. Moisturizing shampoo

B. Bath oil (e.g., Alpha Keri®)

C. Elizabethan collar

D. Benedryl® or diphenhydramine elixir (12.5 mg/ml liquid)

III. First Aid

A. Shampooing the pet will likely provide temporary relief from its symptoms. Use a shampoo for dogs (moisturizing shampoo is best). While restraining the dog, lather the pet and let stand for 15-20 minutes. Rinse well with warm tap water. Next, mix 1 tablespoon of bath oil (e.g., Alpha Keri®) with 2 quarts of warm tap water. Then pour the bath-oil mixture over the dog's coat, being careful not to get any in its eyes. Let the coat dry naturally. Consult your veterinarian for the proper type of shampoo and for specific instructions.

B. If the dog is biting itself, it may be necessary to apply an Elizabethan collar to prevent more damage to the skin. See page 48 on how to make and use an Elizabethan collar.

C. If you are unable to reach a veterinarian, you may give the dog Benedryl® or diphenhydramine elixir (12.5 mg/ml liquid) as follows:

(1) 1/8 teaspoon for dogs weighing less than five pounds.

(2) 1/4 teaspoon for dogs weighing 5 to 20 pounds.

(3) 1/2 teaspoon for dogs weighing 21 to 60 pounds.

(4) 1 teaspoon for dogs weighing more than 60 pounds.

D. Seek veterinary help as soon as possible to give more permanent relief from the allergy.

PROBLEM/CONDITION – ANAL GLAND/SAC ABSCESS

Anal glands/sacs are located along the side of the rectum at the 4 o'clock and 8 o'clock positions. They normally fill with a foul-smelling secretion that is discharged from the glands through small ducts during bowel movements. On occasion, these glands become infected or the ducts become plugged, and the secretion builds. The pressure in the glands becomes so great that the gland and the skin over the area break open and blood, pus and foul discharge may spill out.

I. **Symptoms (some or all may be present)**
A. Scooting butt on floor
B. Swelling around rectum
C. Open wound near rectum
D. Blood, pus or foul discharge under the tail
E. Difficulty sitting
F. Licking the rectum

II. **First-Aid Materials**
A. Muzzle
B. Pet shampoo or moisturizing shampoo
C. Antibiotic ointment (e.g., Polysporin®)

III. **First Aid**
A. You may wish to use a muzzle to prevent being bitten when you treat your dog. However, use a muzzle only if the dog is not having difficulty breathing and has not been vomiting. If at any time the dog has difficulty breathing, remove the muzzle. Also, do not use a muzzle if your dog has a flat face (e.g., a pug, boxer, English bulldog, etc.).
B. Fill a bathtub with warm water, and have the dog sit in the tub for

10 to 20 minutes.

C. If the dog is not in too much pain, cleanse the area under its tail with shampoo, and then rinse well. Dry the dog with a towel.

D. Apply antibiotic ointment (e.g., Polysporin®) to any open wounds.

E. If necessary, apply an Elizabethan collar to prevent the dog from licking its rectum.

F. Contact a veterinarian for additional care.

PROBLEM/CONDITION – ANEMIA

Anemia has many causes, but regardless of the origin of the anemia, the result is an inability of the blood to carry oxygen. Causes of anemia in dogs include flea bites, internal or external bleeding, poisonings, autoimmune diseases, cancers and nutritional deficiencies. It is important that the dog receive proper diagnosis of the condition from a veterinarian so that appropriate treatment can be administered.

I.   Symptoms (some or all may be present)
A.   Listlessness and depression
B.   Pale or white gums
C.   Loss of appetite
D.   Labored breathing
E.   Collapse

II.   First Aid
A.   The dog should see a veterinarian for proper diagnosis as soon as possible.
B.   Minimize stress during handling and transportation.
C.   Feed the dog a balanced dog-diet with an appropriate vitamin supplement prescribed by your veterinarian. Hand feed if necessary.

PROBLEM/CONDITION – ANTIFREEZE TOXICITY

Antifreeze is a common poison to pets for three reasons: it is a commonly-used product; it is often improperly discarded; and it is sweet to the taste.

Antifreeze contains ethylene glycol which, when metabolized, causes kidney damage that is usually fatal. Even a small amount will cause severe illness or death. Because the toxin is rapidly absorbed, symptoms may appear as early as one hour after ingestion. Symptoms are vague and mimic those of many other conditions and diseases.

I. **Symptoms (some or all may be present)**
A. Increased thirst
B. Vomiting and diarrhea
C. Depression
D. Loss of coordination
E. Kidney failure (sometimes preceded by apparent improvement in the dog's condition)

II. **First-Aid Materials**
A. Hydrogen peroxide
B. Liquor (e.g., vodka, whiskey, gin, rum)
C. Eyedropper or dosage syringe

III. **First Aid**
A. If an exposure is suspected, induce vomiting by feeding the dog 1 teaspoon of hydrogen peroxide (mixed with 1 teaspoon milk if available). If the dog will not drink the mixture or if there is no milk available, then force-feed the dog the hydrogen peroxide using an eyedropper or dosage syringe. If vomiting does not occur within 10 minutes, repeat the procedure up to two times.
B. Get immediate veterinary help.

C. If a veterinarian cannot be found, then when vomiting ceases or if vomiting cannot be induced, feed the dog, using an eyedropper or dosage syringe, 2 tablespoons of liquor (e.g., vodka, whiskey, gin, rum) mixed with 2 tablespoons of half and half cream. (If half and half cream is not available, then use milk or water.) Wait 10 minutes, and if there are no signs of depression or intoxication, administer another 1 tablespoon of liquor mixed with 1 tablespoon of half and half cream. (The ethanol in liquor competes with the ethylene glycol metabolism decreasing the amounts that may cause damage to the kidneys. It also promotes increased urination to allow faster excretion of the poison.)

D. Seek veterinary attention for further treatment.

PROBLEM/CONDITION – BACK AND NECK INJURY

Back and neck injury may be the result of a muscle strain, trauma or a variety of other situations. In some instances the injury may be a herniated (slipped) disc or even a tumor near the spine.

I. **Symptoms (some or all may be present)**
A. Restricted or painful movement
B. Difficulty lifting head
C. Lameness
D. Walking hunched-over
E. Depression and loss of appetite
F. Paralysis (if the spinal cord is affected)

II. **First-Aid Materials**
A. Pet carrier (if you have a small dog)
B. Towels
C. Blanket
D. 2-liter soda bottle filled with warm water
E. Muzzle
F. Plywood board cut to fit your dog and your car

III. **First Aid**
A. Seek veterinary advice immediately. Back and neck injuries require professional attention.
B. Restrict the dog's activity. Minimize handling and movement of the dog.
C. If you need to transport your dog, plan the transport carefully to minimize movement of the dog. Use the following procedures to ensure the safest possible transport for your dog:
(1) Because back and neck injuries are painful, you may wish to use a muzzle to prevent being bitten when you move your

dog. However, use a muzzle only if the dog is not having difficulty breathing and has not been vomiting. If at any time the dog has difficulty breathing, remove the muzzle. Also, do not use a muzzle if your dog has a flat face (e.g., a pug, boxer, English bulldog, etc.).

(2) **To transport a small dog**, obtain a pet carrier that has a removable top. If a pet carrier is not available, use a corrugated cardboard box of an appropriate size. A carrier or box that opens at the top rather than the side is preferable because the dog can be put in and taken out without pushing or pulling the pet. Slide your hands under the dog to lift the pet. Take care to support the dog's entire body as you lift and place the dog into the carrier. Place towels around the dog to keep the pet from sliding in the pet carrier. Place a 2-liter soda bottle filled with warm water (not hot water) against the dog. See illustration on page 125.

(3) **To transport a medium-size or large dog**, obtain a plywood board that will fit easily into your car to use as a stretcher. Slide the dog onto the board taking care to move the pet as little as possible. If a board is not available, you may use a blanket or towel as a stretcher instead, but the board is highly preferable because it will result in less movement of the pet and therefore less chance of aggravating the injury. Ideally, place the plywood board with the dog on it into your vehicle. If the board will not fit, slide the dog off of the board and onto the seat with as little movement of the pet as possible. If you have used a blanket or towel rather than a board, keep the blanket or towel under the dog when you put the pet into the car. Pack blankets around the dog to keep the pet warm. If you are concerned that the dog may slide off of the seat onto the floor, pack the floor area with a pillow or blankets. Place one or two 2-liter soda bottles filled with warm water (not hot water) against the dog. See illustrations on pages 125-126.

D.   For more information, see Transportation on pages 26-29.

PROBLEM/CONDITION –
BEE STINGS

When a dog is stung, it is usually stung on an exposed area like the nose or mouth. Fortunately, severe allergic reactions are less common in dogs than in humans.

I. **Symptoms (some or all may be present)**
A. Dog scratching and rubbing the area of the sting
B. Swelling
C. Enlargement of the lips or nose (because most stings are to the face and mouth)
D. Difficulty breathing (though less common in dogs than in people)

II. **First-Aid Materials**
A. Ice
B. Towel
C. Benedryl® or diphenhydramine elixir (12.5 mg/ml liquid)

III. **First Aid**
A. Apply ice wrapped in a towel over the swollen, painful areas.
B. Seek veterinary attention for medication.
C. If you are unable to reach a veterinarian, you may give the dog Benedryl® or diphenhydramine elixir (12.5 mg/ml liquid) as follows:
   (1) 1/8 teaspoon for dogs weighing less than five pounds.
   (2) 1/4 teaspoon for dogs weighing 5 to 20 pounds.
   (3) 1/2 teaspoon for dogs weighing 21 to 60 pounds.
   (4) 1 teaspoon for dogs weighing more than 60 pounds.
D. If there is no improvement within 1 hour after administering medication, or if the condition worsens, seek veterinary assistance.

PROBLEM/CONDITION – BITE WOUNDS

Because of a dog's natural instinct to be territorial and protective, it is common for dogs to fight among themselves and with other animals. Bite wounds are often more serious than they may at first appear because the damage on the surface of the skin is usually less severe than the injury to underlying tissue. When a dog is bitten by another dog, the muscle under the skin is often bruised, crushed or torn, and the wound can be extremely painful. Bite wounds often become infected.

I. Symptoms (some or all may be present)
A. Punctured, torn or lacerated skin with or without bleeding
B. Swelling
C. Painful area
D. Depression, loss of appetite or other signs of illness

II. First-Aid Materials
A. Contact-lens saline solution or water
B. Antibacterial soap
C. Clippers or scissors
D. Antibiotic ointment (e.g., Polysporin®)
E. Wrap material and/or Elizabethan collar

III. First Aid
A. Clip hair away from wound.
B. Cleanse the wound using soap and saline solution or water.
C. Apply antibiotic ointment to the wound.
D. If necessary, apply a wrap over the wound and/or use an Elizabethan collar to keep the dog from licking, scratching or chewing the area. See page 37 on Wrapping a Wound and page 48 on how to make an Elizabethan collar.
E. Seek veterinary help for antibiotic therapy.

PROBLEM/CONDITION – BLEEDING

External bleeding may result from an abrasion or laceration, trauma (e.g., gunshot wound, hit by car), bite wound abscess or compound fracture. Internal bleeding may result from trauma that does not cause a break in the skin, injury to a large muscle mass, a bone fracture, a tumor, toxicity from rat poisoning or injury of an internal organ. Whenever significant bleeding occurs, immediate action is required to prevent shock.

I. **Symptoms (some or all may be present)**
A. Blood coming from a wound
B. Blood accumulating under the skin, looking like a bruise
C. Blood in the dog's urine, feces or vomitus
D. Weakness
E. Pale gums
F. Labored breathing
G. Distended (enlarged) abdomen

II. **First-Aid Materials**
A. Clean towel
B. Gauze sponges
C. Nonstick adhesive tape
D. Nonstick bandages
E. Gauze wrap

III. **First Aid**
A. For internal bleeding:
    (1) Seek veterinary assistance immediately. Internal bleeding is an urgent emergency requiring professional assistance.
    (2) While awaiting veterinary assistance, keep the dog warm by placing a 2-liter soda bottle filled with warm water (not hot

66

water) against the dog. Cover the dog with a towel or blanket.

(3) Monitor the dog's vital signs (temperature, pulse and respirations) every 15 minutes and record the information. Try to keep the dog's temperature within the range of 101-103 degrees Fahrenheit. If the dog's temperature rises above 103 degrees Fahrenheit, remove the warm soda bottle. If the dog's temperature falls below 100 degrees, place an additional warm-water soda bottle against the dog, but make sure the water is not hot and make sure the bottle is against the dog and not on top of or underneath the dog.

B. For external bleeding:

(1) Locate the source of bleeding.

(2) Using a clean towel or gauze sponges, apply direct pressure to the wound for 5-10 minutes.

(3) If the bleeding does not stop, apply a wrap as follows:

a) Press nonstick bandage to wound.

b) Secure nonstick bandage to wound by wrapping gauze around the leg or body. The gauze should be pulled snug but not tight. The wrap tightness should not restrict the dog's circulation or breathing.

c) Secure the gauze by applying adhesive tape to the wrap.

d) Monitor the pet for any evidence of swelling to the limb below the wrap. If swelling occurs, then the wrap is too tight and should be removed immediately. If the dog's breathing is hindered, also remove the wrap.

(4) If the bleeding was difficult to stop, do not attempt to clean the wound or apply antibiotic ointment because the clot may be disrupted and severe hemorrhage may resume.

(5) For future reference, note the amount of blood loss from the injury. If the injury seems severe, treat the dog for shock as follows:

a) Keep the dog warm by placing a 2-liter soda bottle filled with warm water (not hot water) against the dog. Cover the dog with a towel or blanket.

b) Monitor the dog's vital signs (temperature, pulse and respirations) every 15 minutes and record the information. Try to keep the dog's temperature within the range of 100-103 degrees Fahrenheit. If the dog's temperature rises above 103 degrees Fahrenheit, remove the warm soda bottle. If the dog's temperature falls below 100 degrees, place an additional warm-water soda bottle against the dog, but make sure the water is not hot and make sure the bottle is against the dog and not on top of or underneath the dog.

(6) Call your veterinarian immediately. For best healing, lacerations should be repaired as soon as possible (ideally within one hour after the injury). As more time elapses, the wound becomes contaminated and may not be able to be closed.

C. For bleeding from the mouth:

(1) Do not muzzle the dog.

(2) If there is bleeding from the mouth but there is no injury to the mouth, then follow the procedures on page 66 for internal bleeding.

(3) If the outside of the mouth is bleeding, follow the instructions for external bleeding on page 67.

(4) If the dog has lost one or more teeth:

(a) If you can find the teeth, pick them up by the crown (i.e., NOT by the roots) and place them in a cup of milk. The milk will preserve the teeth short-term and may enable your veterinarian to save them.

(b) Seek veterinary assistance immediately.

PROBLEM/CONDITION – BLOAT AND TWISTED STOMACH

When a dog's stomach becomes distended by gas (a condition called "bloat") or when the stomach actually twists and cuts off the blood supply to the stomach (called "twisted stomach", "gastric volvulus" or "gastric torsion"), the result is extreme pain. If the dog does not receive immediate veterinary care, the condition is usually fatal.

Bloat and twisted stomach are conditions of unknown origin. Deep-chested dogs (e.g., Great Danes, St. Bernards, Weimaraners) are more predisposed than others to these conditions. Some veterinarians recommend that deep-chested dogs not be exercised shortly after they have eaten as a precautionary measure for avoiding bloat and twisted stomach.

I. **Symptoms (some or all may be present)**

A. Belching

B. Increased gas noises from abdomen

C. Dry heaves or retching (i.e., unable to vomit)

D. Distended abdomen (usually, but not always)

E. Restlessness or pacing

F. Crying

G. Anxiety followed by depression

H. Collapse

II. **First-Aid Materials**

A. 2-liter soda bottle

B. Blanket or towels

C. Thermometer

III. **First Aid**

A. Contact a veterinarian immediately. The conditions are life-threatening and may require immediate surgery.

B.   Keep the dog warm by placing a 2-liter soda bottle filled with warm water (not hot water) against the dog. See illustration on page 125. Cover the dog with a towel or blanket.

C.   Monitor the dog's vital signs (temperature, pulse and respirations) every 15 minutes and record the information. Try to keep the dog's temperature within the range of 101-103 degrees Fahrenheit. If the dog's temperature rises above 103 degrees Fahrenheit, remove the warm soda bottle. If the dog's temperature falls below 100 degrees, place an additional warm-water soda bottle against the dog, but make sure the water is not hot and make sure the bottle is against the dog and not on top of or underneath the dog. See illustration on page 126.

PROBLEM/CONDITION – BURNS

Many burns are not evident when they occur because the fur often conceals the injury to the skin. However, in some cases the fur will be burned away, and the injury will be readily evident. Burns can result from a variety of sources including chemicals, plants, heat, electricity and hot water. Burns should always be treated as soon as possible.

I. **Symptoms (some or all may be present)**

A. If the fur is still present, the area of the burn may feel like a thickened area under the hair coat.

B. The burned area may feel hardened and may or may not be painful.

C. The pet may lick or scratch at the affected area.

D. If the burn is not recognized early, the fur and skin may start to peel away from the dog's body leaving a deep, weeping sore.

E. Signs of secondary complications include weakness (from dehydration), infections and depression.

II. **First-Aid Materials**

A. Pet shampoo

B. Contact-lens saline solution

C. Antibiotic ointment (e.g., Polysporin®)

III. **First Aid**

A. **If the burn was caused by unknown chemicals,**

   (1) Bathe the dog immediately to remove any remaining chemicals. Use copious amounts of water. If available, use a pet shampoo (lather, let stand for 10 minutes, rinse).

   (2) Rinse the burned area in saline, and then cover the wound

71

with antibiotic ointment. If the dog licks or scratches the area, cover the burn with a wrap. (See Wrapping a Wound on page 37.)

B. **If the burn was caused by an acid,**

    (1) Rinse the area with copious amounts of water.

    (2) Apply a paste of 1 part baking soda to 2 parts water to the affected areas.

C. **If the burn was caused by an alkali,**

    (1) Rinse the area with copious amounts of water.

    (2) Apply a solution of 1 part vinegar to 4 parts water.

D. **If the burn was caused by electricity,**

    (1) Cover the wound with antibiotic ointment. If the dog licks or scratches the area, cover the burn with a wrap. (See Wrapping a Wound on page 37.)

    (2) Seek veterinary assistance immediately because electric shock can cause dangerous arrhythmias (i.e., heart damage).

E. Because burns can have serious side effects like dehydration and secondary infections, it is important to get prompt medical care.

PROBLEM/CONDITION – CHOCOLATE TOXICITY

Chocolate contains a substance called theobromine which cannot be metabolized readily by dogs. Even in small quantities, chocolate may be toxic to your dog.

I. **Symptoms (some or all may be present)**

A. Moderate to severe vomiting and diarrhea

B. Excitability and nervousness

C. Muscle tremors and/or seizures

D. Heart failure

II. **First-Aid Materials**

A. Hydrogen peroxide

B. Eyedropper or dosage syringe

III. **First Aid**

A. Induce vomiting if the ingestion has occurred within the previous 6 hours. To induce vomiting, feed the dog 1 teaspoon of hydrogen peroxide (mixed with 1 teaspoon milk if available). If the dog will not drink the mixture or if there is no milk available, then force-feed the dog the hydrogen peroxide using an eyedropper. If vomiting does not occur in 10 minutes, repeat the procedure twice if needed.

B. See a veterinarian for further monitoring and supportive care.

PROBLEM/CONDITION – CHOKING

It is not normal for a dog to choke on its food. When choking does occur in dogs, it is frequently the result of something being lodged in the dog's mouth that has no business being there (i.e., something other than dog food). Sometimes dogs choke on toys, bones or rawhide. If you give your dog rawhide to chew on, make sure that the rawhide is too large for the pet to swallow, and when it becomes smaller from the dog's chewing, discard it promptly. See the section on Prevention starting on page 12 of this book for some precautions for avoiding choking.

I. Symptoms (some or all may be present)
A. Drooling
B. Pawing at mouth
C. Collapse
D. Labored breathing
E. Anxious behavior

II. First-Aid Materials
A. 1-inch roll of tape
B. Pencil with eraser

III. First Aid
A. Open the dog's mouth to see whether a foreign object is lodged in the dog's mouth or throat, but take care to prevent being bitten. If necessary, use a small roll of first-aid tape as a wedge to keep the dog's mouth open to allow better access and to protect you from the dog's teeth. (See illustration on page 76.)
B. If the dog's airway is not blocked, wait for veterinary assistance before attempting to remove any object; your efforts could do more harm than good. If the airway is blocked, use the eraser end of a pencil to try gently to dislodge the object.

C. If fluid is causing the choking, try wiping the fluid from the mouth using a tissue. You may need to hold the dog with its head lower than its chest for approximately 5 to 10 seconds in order for the fluid to drain. Repeat this process no more than five times.

D. If the pet becomes unconscious:

   (1) Observe for breathing by watching the dog's chest rise and fall.

   (2) **If the dog is breathing**, proceed to Step F; do not use CPR.

E. **If the dog is not breathing**, proceed with CPR as follows:

   (1) Establish an airway by removing any debris from the dog's mouth or by moving the tongue from the back of the throat. (See illustration page 42.) Check for breathing by watching the dog's chest rise and fall. If the dog is breathing, proceed no further; do not use CPR.

   (2) If the dog is not breathing, lay the dog on its side (and throughout these procedures keep the dog on its side). Check for a pulse by placing a hand over the dog's chest just behind the shoulder blade (see page 44) to feel the heartbeat or by placing a hand in the groin area to feel the femoral pulse.

   (3) Cup your hand(s) over the dog's nose and mouth to form a seal. Deliver 1 breath into the pet every 2 seconds. If the seal is proper, you should observe the dog's chest rise and fall.

   (4) If after you have delivered 5 breaths the dog does not show signs of breathing on its own or signs of consciousness, and there is no heartbeat, then have a helper place a hand just behind the dog's shoulder blades (as illustrated on page 44), and apply gentle but firm compressions downward (compressing 1/2 to 1 inch for a small dog up to as much as 2 inches for a large dog) at a rate of 1 compression every 2 seconds. If a helper is not available, alternate delivering 2 breaths then 10 compressions. **Do not do any compressions if there is a pulse, no matter how faint.**

   (5) Check for a pulse and breathing every 2 minutes. If there is

no pulse and breathing, continue for up to 10 minutes before giving up.

F. Sedation may be necessary to remove a foreign object; if your attempt at home is unsuccessful, seek immediate veterinary care.

G. Regardless of whether the object has been removed, have your dog checked by a veterinarian as soon as possible for lacerations in the mouth and throat.

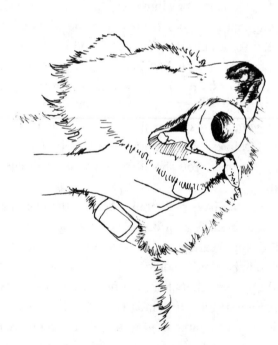

PROBLEM/CONDITION – COLITIS

Colitis is inflammation of the colon. It has many different causes including allergic reactions, dietary indiscretions, foreign bodies, parasitic infestations and cancers. Even though not all causes of colitis are serious, the amount of discomfort the dog feels warrants the classification of colitis as an emergency.

I. **Symptoms (some or all may be present)**

A. Blood or mucous in the stool

B. Soft stools – If bowel movements cannot be observed, check under the dog's tail for stool pasted to the fur.

C. Foreign material (e.g., string, grass, panty hose, socks, etc.) protruding from the rectum – **Do not pull on these objects because they could tear or cut the bowels.**

D. Straining – (Note, however, that straining may be the result of a life-threatening urinary blockage. Watch to make sure the dog urinates.)

II. **First Aid**

A. If there is no foreign object protruding from the rectum and there are no signs of illness other than colitis, withhold food for 4 hours. (This time reference is for a normal, otherwise healthy, adult dog. Puppies and old dogs should not be restricted from food for more than a couple of hours.) DO NOT withhold water unless your dog is vomiting. If there are other symptoms of illness, such as vomiting, lack of appetite or listlessness, contact a veterinarian immediately. If your dog has no symptoms of other illness but is not more comfortable within 4 hours, contact a veterinarian. Many times colitis requires treatment with antibiotics or anti-inflammatories.

B. If any foreign object (e.g., grass, string, cloth, etc.) is protruding from the rectum, do not pull on the object; it could lacerate the bowels. Instead, if the object is protruding more than four inches, cut the object with a scissors (to within four inches of the rectum) taking care not to cut the dog. Contact a veterinarian immediately.

C. Add 1-2 teaspoons of bran flakes to your dog's meals to increase the fiber in your pet's diet or obtain a prescription food from your veterinarian.

D. To aid your dog's digestion, feed your dog more frequently but in smaller portions.

PROBLEM/CONDITION – CONSTIPATION

Dogs rarely become constipated, but when they do, causes include dehydration, perianal hernias, prostatic enlargement and foreign bodies in the digestive tract. Note, however, that a dog that strains to have a bowel movement is not necessarily constipated. (See Colitis on page 77, Straining on page 175, and Urinary-Tract Irritations on page 140.)

I.   **Symptoms (some or all may be present)**

A.   Lack of bowel movement within 48 hours

B.   Straining to go to the bathroom

C.   Loss of appetite

II. **First-Aid Materials**

A.   Bran flakes

B.   Mineral oil

III. **First Aid**

A.   If the dog is uncomfortable or if more than 2 days have passed since a bowel movement, contact your veterinarian.

B.   Most dogs do not tolerate home enemas. An enema should be performed by a professional because a dog can be injured easily if it struggles during the process.

C.   Feed the dog 2 tablespoons of bran flakes with each meal.

D.   Encourage the dog to drink water.

E.   Mix 1/4 teaspoon mineral oil into the dog's food to soften the dog's stools.

PROBLEM/CONDITION – CORONAVIRUS

Coronavirus is similar to parvovirus in that the disease attacks the lining of the digestive tract causing vomiting and bloody diarrhea. Coronavirus infections tend to be slightly less severe than parvovirus but are still often fatal when not treated. Coronavirus is a highly contagious disease. It affects young, small and debilitated dogs most severely. Death is usually due to dehydration or overwhelming infection that spreads to the blood. Dogs that are infected with the virus can be contagious to other dogs for two weeks, and the virus can remain in the environment for years; proper disinfecting is required to ensure that healthy dogs entering the same environment do not become infected.

Vaccinations can prevent this disease. Consult your veterinarian regarding vaccinations and other precautions.

I.   Symptoms (some or all may be present)

A.   Loss of appetite

B.   Depression

C.   Vomiting

D.   Watery diarrhea that is often bloody and usually foul-smelling

E.   Pale gums

F.   Shivering

G.   Rapid decline in physical condition

H.   Collapse

II.   First-Aid Materials

A.   Kaopectate®

B.   Eyedropper or dosage syringe

C.   Boiled hamburger and plain cooked rice

III.   First Aid

A.   Seek veterinary care immediately. Coronavirus is often fatal.

B. If there is no vomiting, feed the dog Kaopectate® using an eyedropper or dosage syringe:
   (1) 1 to 2 teaspoons for dogs weighing less than 20 pounds,
   (2) 3 to 4 teaspoons for dogs weighing 20 or more pounds.
C. Repeat Step B every 4 to 6 hours for adult dogs and every 2 to 4 hours for puppies less than 14 weeks old.
D. Withhold food for 2-4 hours if diarrhea is present and if there is no other symptom of illness. Withhold both food and water if the dog is also vomiting, but do not withhold water for more than 2 hours. Do not withhold water if the dog is not vomiting. The time period for withholding food should be based on whether your pet is a normal, healthy adult versus a puppy, an elderly dog or a dog with any special or compromising conditions. If your dog has diabetes or any other type of illness or medical condition, consult your veterinarian first before withholding food and water.
E. When you do resume feeding your dog, the best home remedy for diarrhea is to prepare a 50/50 mixture of boiled hamburger (drain off the water and fat) and plain cooked rice. Appropriate feedings are as follows:
   (1) 1/4 cup of the mixture 4 times per day for small dogs,
   (2) 1/2 cup of the mixture 4 times per day for medium dogs,
   (3) 3/4 cup of the mixture 4 times per day for large dogs.
   Your veterinarian may wish to adjust the servings or may recommend a prescription diet instead.
F. Note the frequency and substance of the diarrhea.
G. Coronavirus is often fatal, and professional veterinary care is critical for your dog's survival. The above procedures are appropriate while waiting for professional help, but they are not sufficient to save your dog.

PROBLEM/CONDITION – DIARRHEA

The goal in helping a dog with diarrhea is to comfort the pet and lessen the symptoms until the cause can be determined. There are many causes of diarrhea including infections, dietary changes, foreign bodies, parasites and poisons.

I.   Symptoms (some or all may be present)

A.   Soft to watery stools

B.   Loss of appetite

C.   Painful abdomen

II.   First-Aid Materials

A.   Kaopectate®

B.   Eyedropper or dosage syringe

C.   Boiled hamburger and plain cooked rice

III.   First Aid

A.   If there is no vomiting, feed the dog Kaopectate® using an eyedropper or dosage syringe:

   (1)   1 to 2 teaspoons for dogs weighing less than 20 pounds,

   (2)   3 to 4 teaspoons for dogs weighing 20 or more pounds.

B.   Repeat Step A every 4 to 6 hours for adult dogs and every 2 to 4 hours for puppies less than 14 weeks old.

C.   Withhold food for 2-4 hours if diarrhea is present and if there is no other symptom of illness. Withhold both food and water if the dog is also vomiting, but do not withhold water for more than 2 hours. Do not withhold water if the dog is not vomiting. The time period for withholding food should be based on whether your pet is a normal, healthy adult versus a puppy, an elderly dog or a dog with any special or compromising conditions. If your dog has diabetes or any other type of illness or medical condition, consult your veterinarian first before withholding food and water.

D. When you do resume feeding your dog, the best home remedy for diarrhea is to prepare a 50/50 mixture of boiled hamburger (drain off the water and fat) and plain cooked rice. Appropriate feedings are as follows:

(1) 1/4 cup of the mixture 4 times per day for small dogs,

(2) 1/2 cup of the mixture 4 times per day for medium dogs,

(3) 3/4 cup of the mixture 4 times per day for large dogs.

Your veterinarian may wish to adjust the servings or may recommend a prescription diet instead.

E. Note the frequency and substance of the diarrhea.

F. If symptoms persist for more than 4 hours, or if they worsen or return, contact the pet's doctor immediately.

PROBLEM/CONDITION – DIGESTIVE UPSET

The goal in helping a dog with digestive upset is to comfort the pet and lessen the symptoms until the cause can be determined. There are many causes of digestive upset, including infections, dietary changes, foreign bodies, parasites, and poisons. Never feed a dog bones or table scraps.

I.   **Symptoms (some or all may be present)**
A.   Loss of appetite
B.   Soft to watery stools
C.   Painful abdomen
D.   Vomiting

II. **First-Aid Materials**
A.   Kaopectate®
B.   Eyedropper or dosage syringe
C.   Boiled hamburger and plain cooked rice

III. **First Aid**
A.   If there is no vomiting, feed the dog Kaopectate® using an eyedropper or dosage syringe:
     (1) 1 to 2 teaspoons for dogs weighing less than 20 pounds,
     (2) 3 to 4 teaspoons for dogs weighing 20 or more pounds.
B.   Repeat Step A every 4 to 6 hours for adult dogs and every 2 to 4 hours for puppies less than 14 weeks old.
C.   Withhold food for 2-4 hours if diarrhea is present and if there is no other symptom of illness. Withhold both food and water if the dog is also vomiting, but do not withhold water for more than 2 hours. Do not withhold water if the dog is not vomiting. The time period for withholding food should be based on whether your pet is a normal, healthy adult versus a puppy, an elderly dog

or a dog with any special or compromising conditions. (If your cat has diabetes or any other type of illness or medical condition, consult your veterinarian first before withholding food and water.)

D. When you do resume feeding your dog, the best home remedy for diarrhea is to prepare a 50/50 mixture of boiled hamburger (drain off the water and fat) and plain cooked rice. Appropriate feedings are as follows:

(1) 1/4 cup of the mixture 4 times per day for small dogs,

(2) 1/2 cup of the mixture 4 times per day for medium dogs,

(3) 3/4 cup of the mixture 4 times per day for large dogs.

Your veterinarian may wish to adjust the servings or may recommend a prescription diet instead.

E. Note the frequency and substance of the diarrhea.

F. If symptoms persist for more than 4 hours, or if they worsen or return, contact the pet's doctor immediately.

PROBLEM/CONDITION – DROWNING

Dogs that love to swim or ride in boats or live near any body of water, including flood plains, are at risk of drowning. While most dogs are natural swimmers, some are more proficient than others, and waves, undertows or fast moving water may be more than your dog can handle.

I. Symptoms (one or both may be present)

A. Witnessing the event

B. Finding the dog collapsed on a shoreline

II. First Aid

A. Hold the dog upside-down by its hind legs to allow the water and fluid to drain from its airway. Gently pounding the dog's chest may hasten fluid removal.

B. Check for breathing by watching the dog's chest rise and fall.

C. **If the dog is breathing**, proceed to Step E. Do not use CPR.

D. **If the dog is not breathing,**

    (1) Establish an airway by removing any debris from the dog's mouth or by moving the tongue from the back of the throat. (See illustration page 42.) Check for breathing by watching the dog's chest rise and fall. If the dog is breathing, proceed no further, and do not use CPR.

    (2) If the dog is not breathing, lay the dog on its side (and throughout these procedures keep the dog on its side). Check for a pulse by placing a hand over the dog's chest just behind the shoulder blade (see page 44) to feel the heartbeat or by placing a hand in the groin area to feel the femoral pulse.

    (3) Cup your hand(s) over the dog's nose and mouth to form a

seal. Deliver 1 breath into the pet every 2 seconds. If the seal is proper, you should observe the dog's chest rise and fall.

(4) If after you have delivered 5 breaths the dog does not show signs of breathing on its own or signs of consciousness, and there is no heartbeat, then have a helper place a hand just behind the dog's shoulder blades (as illustrated on page 44), and apply gentle but firm compressions downward (compressing 1/2 to 1 inch for a small dog up to as much as 2 inches for a large dog) at a rate of 1 compression every 2 seconds. If a helper is not available, alternate delivering 2 breaths then 10 compressions. **Do not do any compressions if there is a pulse, no matter how faint.**

(5) Check for a pulse and breathing every 2 minutes. If there is no pulse and breathing, continue for up to 10 minutes before giving up.

E. Seek veterinary help for treatment to remove residual fluid, treat for infection and monitor the dog's condition.

PROBLEM/CONDITION – EYE EMERGENCIES

Examples of eye emergencies include corneal scratches, glaucoma, contusions, corneal ulcers, foreign debris in the eyes and popped-out (proptosed) eyes. A delay in treatment may result in permanent loss of vision.

I. Symptoms (some or all may be present)
A. Squinting
B. Excessive tearing (may be clear or cloudy)
C. Dog rubbing its eye(s) with its paw or rubbing its face on the ground
D. Enlarged eye(s)
E. Reddened white of the eye(s)

II. First-Aid Materials
A. Contact-lens saline solution

III. First Aid
A. If the irritation is minor, gently rinse the eye(s) with the contact-lens saline solution by applying several drops to the affected eye(s). This may dislodge any foreign debris causing the irritation. If the irritation is serious, contact professional help immediately.
B. If the symptoms persist, worsen or improve but then reappear, call the dog's veterinarian.
C. To keep the dog from further injuring the eye, apply an Elizabethan collar. (See page 48.)
D. Never apply human medicine to a pet's eye without the consent of a veterinarian.

PROBLEM/CONDITION – FISH HOOKS

Fish hooks are an obvious hazard if your dog is nearby when anyone is fishing. In addition, dogs sometimes scavenge through storage areas where they are drawn to hooks and lures and often chew on them because of residual odors from the fish or bait. Often hooks become lodged in a dog's lips or feet.

I. Symptoms (some or all may be present)

A. Portion of hook lodged in skin

B. Pawing at mouth or salivating

C. Limping

II. First-Aid Materials

A. Muzzle

B. Elizabethan collar

C. Wire cutters

D. Protective eye wear

E. Antibiotic ointment (e.g., Polysporin®)

III. First Aid

A. **If the hook has entered past the barb, do not try to pull the fish hook out of the dog.** The barb will cause severe tearing.

B. If the dog has swallowed the hook and there is fishing line extending outside the dog's mouth, do not pull on the line. Cut the line 6 inches from the dog's mouth, and try to keep the dog from swallowing the end of the line. Seek veterinary help immediately to have the hook extracted.

C. If the hook is lodged somewhere other than the dog's mouth, apply a muzzle to the dog. (Except never muzzle a dog that may have difficulty breathing, has a flat face or small nostrils, or is vomiting.)

D. If the hook is in the dog's mouth, apply an Elizabethan collar to prevent the dog from pawing at the hook.

E. If the hook has not gone all the way through, it will need to be extracted by a veterinarian to minimize damage.

F. If the hook has gone all the way through and is sticking out the other side past the barb, use wire cutters to cut the back end of the hook, and then extract the hook by moving it through the rest of the way. Make sure you use protective eye wear before cutting the hook. Do not try to cut off the barb and back the hook out the way it went in because many hooks have secondary barbs that you might not see, and the secondary barbs can cause severe tearing.

G. After the hook has been removed, clean the wound with soap and water, and apply antibiotic ointment. If the wound is in the bottom of the foot, apply a wrap. See Wrapping a Wound on page 37.

H. Even if you have been successful at removing the hook and cleaning the wound, have your dog checked by a veterinarian as soon as possible.

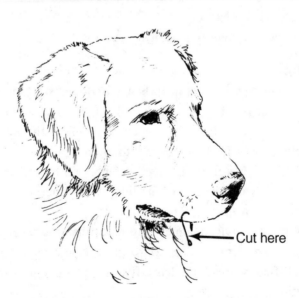

Cut here

PROBLEM/CONDITION – FRACTURES

    The most common cause of fractures is trauma. Regardless of the cause, the single most important thing you can do to help the dog is RESTRICT ACTIVITY. By restricting activity immediately, you decrease the chances of the pet worsening the injury.

    Many fractures are the result of severe trauma, such as getting hit by a car. An emergency involving a fracture should be treated with great urgency because the pet may have life-threatening internal injuries not immediately evident. If a fracture is compound (open to the air) or severely fragmented, the pet can hemorrhage and quickly go into shock.

I.   Symptoms (some or all may be present)

A.   Dogs usually will not bear weight on a fractured leg.

B.   Limbs may appear swollen.

C.   Fractures are usually painful and do not improve with time.

D.   Fractures of the ribs may be associated with difficult breathing.

II.   First-Aid Materials

A.   Gauze sponges and roll gauze

B.   Tape

C.   Muzzle

D.   Towels

E.   Blanket

F.   2-liter soda bottle filled with warm water

G.   Plywood board cut to fit your dog and your car

III.   First Aid

A.   Because fractures are painful, you may wish to use a muzzle to prevent being bitten when you move your dog. However, use a muzzle only if the dog is not having difficulty breathing and has not been vomiting. If at any time the dog has difficulty breathing, remove the muzzle. Also, do not use a muzzle if your dog has a flat face (e.g., a pug, boxer, English bulldog, etc.).

B.   Keep the dog still. If necessary, wrap the pet in a towel or blanket to restrict its movements.

C.   Keep any open wounds covered with gauze and secure with tape.

D.   If an open wound is bleeding profusely, apply pressure over that area.

E.   Seek veterinary help immediately. Plan the transportation to the veterinarian carefully to minimize movement of the dog.

   (1)   **To transport a small dog**, obtain a pet carrier that has a removable top. If a pet carrier is not available, use a corrugated cardboard box of an appropriate size. A carrier or box that opens at the top rather than the side is preferable because the dog can be put in and taken out without pushing or pulling the pet. Slide your hands under the dog to lift the pet. Take care to support the dog's entire body as you lift. Place the dog into the carrier with its injured side up, if possible. Place towels around the dog to keep the pet from sliding in the pet carrier. Place a 2-liter soda bottle filled with warm water (not hot water) against the dog. See illustration on page 125.

   (2)   **To transport a medium-size or large dog**, if the dog cannot walk, obtain a plywood board that will fit easily into your car to use as a stretcher. Slide the dog onto the board taking care to move the pet as little as possible. If a board is not available, you may use a blanket or towel as a stretcher instead, but the board is highly preferable because it will result in less movement of the pet and therefore less chance of aggravating the injury. Ideally, place the plywood board with the dog on it into your vehicle. If the board will not fit, slide the dog off of the board and onto the seat with as little movement of the pet as possible. If you have used a blanket or towel rather than a board, keep the blanket or towel under the dog when you put the pet into the car. Pack blankets around the dog to keep the pet warm. If you are concerned

that the dog may slide off of the seat onto the floor, pack the floor area with a pillow or blankets. Place one or two 2-liter soda bottles filled with warm water (not hot water) against the dog. See illustrations on pages 125-126.

F.   Monitor the dog's vital signs (temperature, pulse and respirations).

G.   Observe for other injuries.

PROBLEM/CONDITION – FROSTBITE

A dog's coat will not protect it from extreme cold. When temperatures or windchill fall below freezing, it is important that your dog has shelter. As with people, frostbite occurs when the extreme cold restricts blood flow to an appendage and thereby causes the tissue to die. The damage is frequently permanent. Frostbite may involve any appendage, but in dogs most often it affects the tips of the ears. Exposure that causes frostbite can also cause death by freezing.

I. Symptoms (one or both may be present)

A. The ears or appendages may appear reddened and blistered. The symptoms may not be evident immediately after exposure to cold but will appear in a short period of time.

B. Frostbitten tissue will eventually turn dark and slough or scar.

II. First-Aid Materials

A. Contact-lens saline solution

B. Antibiotic ointment (e.g., Polysporin®)

C. 2-liter soda bottle

III. First Aid

A. If frostbite is suspected, immediately warm the ears or extremities in tepid water. Do not use hot water.

B. If damage has already occurred, gently rinse the affected area in saline or water and apply antibiotic ointment.

C. If the dog is chilled (hypothermic), fill a 2-liter soda bottle with warm water (not hot water), and place the bottle against the dog as illustrated on page 125. See page 104 for further information and instruction regarding hypothermia.

D. Contact the dog's veterinarian for further instructions.

PROBLEM/CONDITION – HEART DISEASE

Heart disease is a common occurrence in dogs. The disease may be a result of a birth defect, heartworm disease, infection, heart muscle disease, valve disease, or aging. Regardless of the cause, the condition may be very debilitating. Recognizing symptoms early and getting help as soon as possible will increase the dog's comfort level and improve the outcome.

I. Symptoms (some or all may be present)
A. Coughing
B. Labored respirations (or gasping)
C. Weakness
D. Blue-tinged gums or tongue
E. Enlarged abdomen
F. Accelerated or depressed heart rate
G. Loss of consciousness

II. First-Aid Materials
A. Two 2-liter soda bottles
B. Blanket

III. First Aid
A. If the pet is unconscious and does not have a heartbeat or is not breathing, begin CPR immediately:
   (1) Lay the dog on its side (and throughout these procedures keep the dog on its side).
   (2) Check for breathing by watching the dog's chest rise and fall.
   (3) **If the dog is breathing,** proceed to Step B. Do not use CPR.
   (4) **If the dog is not breathing,**

95

a) Establish an airway by removing any debris from the dog's mouth or by moving the tongue from the back of the throat. (See illustration page 42.) Check for breathing by watching the dog's chest rise and fall. If the dog is breathing, proceed to Step B, and do not use CPR.

b) Check for a pulse by placing a hand over the dog's chest just behind the shoulder blade to feel the heartbeat or by placing a hand in the groin area to feel the femoral pulse.

(5) **If the dog still is not breathing,**

a) Cup your hand(s) over the dog's nose and mouth to form a seal. Deliver 1 breath into the pet every 2 seconds. If the seal is proper, you should observe the dog's chest rise and fall.

b) If after you have delivered 5 breaths the dog does not show signs of breathing on its own or signs of consciousness, and there is no heartbeat, then have a helper place a hand just behind the dog's shoulder blades (as illustrated on page 44), and apply gentle but firm compressions downward (compressing 1/2 to 1 inch for a small dog up to as much as 2 inches for a large dog) at a rate of 1 compression every 2 seconds. If a helper is not available, alternate delivering 2 breaths then 10 compressions. **Do not do any compressions if there is a pulse, no matter how faint.**

c) Check for a pulse and breathing every 2 minutes. If there is no pulse and breathing, continue for up to 10 minutes before giving up.

B. Keep the dog calm. Do not use excessive restraint or move the dog more than necessary.

C. Keep the dog warm with the blanket and with the 2-liter soda bottles filled with warm water placed against the dog's body.

D. Call your veterinarian.

PROBLEM/CONDITION – HEAT STROKE OR HYPERTHERMIA

Heat stroke is a common occurrence during the warmer months of the year. Dogs are prone to overheating because they do not sweat. Other factors such as obesity, advanced age, infancy and poor ventilation also predispose dogs to hyperthermia.

I. **Symptoms (some or all may be present)**

A. Panting

B. Weakness or collapse

C. Elevated temperature (from 105 to 110 degrees Fahrenheit)

D. Vomiting, diarrhea and/or lack of urine production

E. Seizures

II. **First-Aid Materials**

A. 2-liter soda bottle

B. Towel

C. Thermometer

III. **First Aid**

A. Take the dog's temperature.

B. If temperature is greater than 106 degrees, immerse the dog in cold water.

C. Monitor the dog's temperature every 2 minutes to observe any change.

D. Stop the cooling process once the dog's temperature drops to 104 degrees. Do not wait until the temperature falls to normal because the dog's temperature may continue to drop.

E. If the temperature falls below 100 degrees Fahrenheit, keep the pet warm by covering it with a towel and by placing a 2-liter soda bottle filled with warm water (not hot water) against the dog.

F. Contact a veterinarian immediately to prevent shock and other complications.

PROBLEM/CONDITION – HIT BY CAR

      In a situation involving serious trauma, such as being hit by a car, immediate care may be crucial to the eventual outcome. In addition to the damage caused by the physical impact, there is a high risk that the animal will go into shock. If your dog is not found by the road after being hit by a car, it may arrive home showing a varying degree of symptoms.

I. Symptoms (some or all may be present)

A. Weakness

B. Lameness

C. Difficulty breathing

D. Bleeding

E. Pale or purple gums

F. Collapse

II. First-Aid Materials

A. Blanket and/or towels

B. Gauze

C. Tape

D. Muzzle

E. Contact-lens saline solution

F. Antibiotic ointment (e.g., Polysporin®)

G. Plywood board cut to fit your dog and your car

III. First Aid

A. If the dog is having difficulty breathing, keep it upright and do not apply any unnecessary or overly-restrictive restraint.

    Because fractures are painful, you may wish to use a muzzle to prevent being bitten when you move your dog. However, use a muzzle only if the dog is not having difficulty breathing and has not been vomiting. If at any time the dog has difficulty breathing, remove the muzzle. Also, do not use a muzzle if your dog has a flat face (e.g., a pug, boxer, English bulldog, etc.).

B.   Keep the dog still. If necessary, wrap the pet in a towel or blanket to restrict its movements.

C.   If an open wound is bleeding profusely, apply pressure over that area. Do not attempt to wash the wound and do not apply any ointment.

D.   Seek veterinary help immediately. Plan the transportation to the veterinarian carefully to minimize movement of the dog.

(1) **To transport a small dog,** obtain a pet carrier that has a removable top. If a pet carrier is not available, use a corrugated cardboard box of an appropriate size. A carrier or box that opens at the top rather than the side is preferable because the dog can be put in and taken out without pushing or pulling the pet. Slide your hands under the dog to lift the pet. Take care to support the dog's entire body as you lift. Place the dog into the carrier with its injured side up, if possible. Place towels around the dog to keep the pet from sliding in the pet carrier. Place a 2-liter soda bottle filled with warm water (not hot water) against the dog. See illustration on page 125.

(2) **To transport a medium-size or large dog,** if the dog cannot walk, obtain a plywood board that will fit easily into your car to use as a stretcher. Slide the dog onto the board taking care to move the pet as little as possible. If a board is not available, you may use a blanket or towel as a stretcher instead, but the board is highly preferable because it will result in less movement of the pet and therefore less chance of aggravating the injury. Ideally, place the plywood board with the dog on it into your vehicle. If the board will not fit, slide the dog off of the board and onto the seat with as little movement of the pet as possible. If you have used a blanket or towel rather than a board, keep the blanket or towel under

the dog when you put the pet into the car. Pack blankets around the dog to keep the pet warm. If you are concerned that the dog may slide off of the seat onto the floor, pack the floor area with a pillow or blankets. Place one or two 2-liter soda bottles filled with warm water (not hot water) against the dog. See illustrations on pages 125-126.

E.   For minor wounds, while awaiting veterinary care, wash with water or saline solution, apply antibiotic ointment and cover with a gauze bandage. If there are other serious injuries, do not treat minor wounds if it will delay other medical attention.

F.   For additional information and instruction about specific injuries, see the appropriate section(s) of this book (e.g., fractures, bleeding, wound care, lacerations, wrapping a wound).

PROBLEM/CONDITION –
HOT SPOTS
(ACUTE MOIST DERMATITIS)

Hot spots, also called acute moist dermatitis, is a common skin disorder that occurs in all breeds of dogs. Hot spots initially appear as reddened areas on the skin that are extremely painful and itchy to the dog. Typically, the dog will lick and chew at the hot spot areas until the hair is missing and the area is raw or bloody. Fleas and/or allergies may make the condition even worse.

I. Symptoms (some or all may be present)
A. Red area under hair or on skin
B. Dog licking or chewing at skin
C. Pain over affected area
D. Hair loss or hair may be sticky

II. First-Aid Materials
A. Scissors
B. Domeboro® tablets/powder packets
C. Antibiotic ointment (e.g., Polysporin®)

III. First Aid
A. Because hot spots are painful, you may wish to use a muzzle to prevent being bitten when you treat your dog. However, use a muzzle only if the dog is not having difficulty breathing and has not been vomiting. If at any time the dog has difficulty breathing, remove the muzzle. Also, do not use a muzzle if your dog has a flat face (e.g., a pug, boxer, English bulldog, etc.).
B. Carefully trim the hair away from affected areas with scissors.
C. Mix 2 tablets or 2 packets of Domeboro® with 2 cups of water.
D. Saturate a cloth with the Domeboro® mixture and apply over the

hot spots for 15 to 30 minutes. Apply antibiotic ointment after the Domeboro® application.

E.   Repeat the application of the Domeboro® mixture, followed by the antibiotic ointment, every 6 to 8 hours.

F.   If the dog persists in licking or chewing the affected areas, apply an Elizabethan collar.

G.   Seek veterinary attention for medication.

PROBLEM/CONDITION – HYPOTHERMIA

Hypothermia (i.e., chilling) is a condition caused by exposure to cold. It may or may not be accompanied by frostbite. If your dog goes outdoors in cold weather, it is important that the pet has adequate shelter (e.g., a barn or a garage). Also note that your dog's general health, age, and build may make the pet more susceptible to hypothermia. Never let your dog outside if the temperature falls below 25 degrees Fahrenheit. Even in temperatures above freezing, your dog can become hypothermic if there is wind and rain. If left untreated, hypothermia can be fatal.

I. Symptoms (some or all may be present)

A. In early stages the dog may be shivering.

B. In later stages the dog will become stuporous, depressed, confused or even comatose.

C. The body temperature will fall below 99 degrees Fahrenheit.

II. First-Aid Materials

A. Thermometer

B. 2-liter soda bottles

C. Towels and/or blanket

III. First Aid

A. Bring the dog into the house or into some other warm area.

B. Take the dog's temperature.

C. If the temperature is below 98 degrees Fahrenheit, rewarm the dog carefully by placing a 2-liter soda bottle filled with warm water against the dog's body. (See illustration on page 125.)

D. Check the dog's temperature every 5-10 minutes. Keep the dog warm by keeping it covered with a blanket, even if its temperature returns to normal.

E. Because there is a danger of shock, immediately seek veterinary care.

PROBLEM/CONDITION – IBUPROFEN TOXICITY

Ibuprofen is an anti-inflammatory drug that, for dogs, is toxic. Because ibuprofen is a common household medication, dogs often have easy access to the drug. Some ibuprofen brands are sugar-coated and appeal to dogs. Human medications should never be given to pets without the advice of a veterinarian.

I. **Symptoms (some or all may be present)**

A. Digestive upset

B. Bloody stool

C. Depression

D. Staggering

E. Increased thirst

F. Increased frequency of urination

G. Liver disease

H. Kidney disease

I. Seizures

II. **First-Aid Materials**

A. Hydrogen peroxide

B. Eyedropper or dosage syringe

III. **First Aid**

A. If the pet is conscious, induce vomiting immediately by feeding the dog 1 teaspoon of hydrogen peroxide (mixed with 1 teaspoon of milk if available). If the dog will not drink the mixture or if there is no milk available, then force-feed the dog the hydrogen peroxide using an eyedropper or dosage syringe. If vomiting does not occur within 10 minutes, repeat the procedure twice.

B. Contact your veterinarian for further treatment regardless of whether you have been successful at inducing vomiting.

PROBLEM/CONDITION – INNER EAR OR VESTIBULAR DISEASE

The inner ear and vestibular system help control balance, posture and head position. Any injury, infection or inflammation in the ear can cause stroke-like symptoms. Early treatment is critical to prevent further damage and possible infection.

I. Symptoms (some or all may be present)
A. Tilted head
B. Disorientation/confusion
C. Stumbling and loss of coordination or balance
D. Walking in circles
E. Eyes involuntarily moving from side to side

II. First-Aid Materials
A. Cotton balls

III. First Aid
A. Look in the ear to see if there is a discharge or something blocking the ear canal. Gently wipe any debris from the ear canal using a cotton ball. If the debris is difficult to remove, seek veterinary assistance to prevent further damage and infection.
B. If the dog is disoriented or appears to have a loss of balance or coordination, block off stairways and restrict the pet's activity. Carry or help the dog out to go to the bathroom four times per day.
C. If the dog shows no sign of nausea, offer food and water by hand feeding; the dog's condition may prevent it from eating and drinking out of a bowl.
D. Seek veterinary care as soon as possible.

PROBLEM/CONDITION – INSECT INGESTION

Many varieties of insects can cause illness from ingestion. The symptoms will vary depending upon the type of insect, the quantity ingested, and the susceptibility of the particular dog. Because of the wide variety of insects, it is impossible to specifically identify which ones are toxic. In general, however, poisoning from insect ingestion is not a problem, and in particular, ingestion of an occasional fly, mosquito or lightning bug is typically harmless. There are some insects that have developed toxicity as part of their evolution to protect themselves from being eaten (e.g., the monarch butterfly), but these are the exceptions. Frequently with insect ingestion the risk of bites and stings in the dog's mouth is greater than the danger from ingestion.

I.   Symptoms (some or all may be present)

A.   Salivation from mouth irritation (from bites or stings)

B.   Weakness

C.   Vomiting

D.   Diarrhea

E.   Disorientation

F.   Difficulty breathing

G.   Seizures

II.   First-Aid Materials

A.   Hydrogen peroxide

B.   Eyedropper

III.   First Aid

A.   If it appears that the dog's mouth is irritated (e.g., if the dog is salivating or rubbing its mouth), flush the dog's mouth with fresh water using an eyedropper.

B.   If the pet shows any signs of illness from ingestion, immediately induce vomiting (unless the dog is unconscious or in a stupor) by feeding the dog 1 teaspoon of hydrogen peroxide (mixed with 1 teaspoon milk if available). If the dog will not drink the mixture or if there is no milk available, then force-feed the dog the hydrogen peroxide using an eyedropper. If vomiting does not occur within 10 minutes, repeat the procedure twice. Seek veterinary assistance for additional care.

C. If possible, identify the type of insect (to assist in appropriate veterinary treatment).

PROBLEM/CONDITION – LOCKED DOGS

When dogs breed, it is normal for them to become locked together during copulation. This occurs because the bulb of the dog's penis enlarges and the female dog's vulva locks around it. Copulation may take up to 20 minutes for completion.

I. Symptoms (one or both may be present)

A. Male dog and female dog unable to separate after copulation.

B. Male and female dog may be connected tail to tail when the male dog dismounts.

II. First Aid

A. Do nothing. Do not disturb or try to separate the animals. Dogs that are forced apart may experience damage to their genitalia. The dogs will eventually separate on their own.

B. Unless you want to have puppies, spay or neuter your dog.

PROBLEM/CONDITION – LUNG DISEASE AND RESPIRATORY DISTRESS

A dog suffering from lung disease or respiratory distress does not receive enough oxygen to be comfortable or function normally. The condition may be caused by many disease processes including pneumonia, trauma, heart disease, heartworm disease and cancer. The condition is life-threatening; contact a veterinarian immediately.

I. **Symptoms (some or all may be present)**

A. The dog may take short, shallow or rapid breaths or may pant.

B. The dog's gum or tongue color may be purple, blue, or pale.

C. The pet may be able only to sit upright with its elbows pointed outward; the dog may not be able to lie flat.

D. The dog may be depressed, but sometimes restless, due to the lack of oxygen.

II. **First Aid**

A. Avoid all stress. The least amount of stress may precipitate a crisis when the pet cannot breathe properly.

B. Do not monitor vital signs.

C. Plan the handling of the dog to minimize excitement. Never hold the dog tightly.

D. Keep the dog in an upright position (i.e., belly down). Never lay the dog on its back or side because those positions make breathing more difficult by putting extra pressure on the chest.

E. Contact a veterinarian immediately.

PROBLEM/CONDITION – PARALYSIS

Paralysis, when it occurs, typically involves the loss of function of the dog's leg(s). Paralysis may or may not be accompanied by numbness. Causes include trauma, herniated disc disease, infections and cancers. Most often paralysis is associated with some type of damage to the spinal cord. To avoid causing additional injury to the spinal cord, it is important to restrict the dog's activity and to disturb the dog as little as possible during transport to a veterinarian.

I.   Symptoms (some or all may be present)

A.   Dragging one or more legs or toes

B.   Back or neck pain

C.   Reluctance to move

D.   Disorientation

E.   Partial or complete loss of the ability to move

II.   First-Aid Materials

A.   Muzzle

B.   Blanket or plywood board (cut to fit your dog and your car)

III.   First Aid

A.   Paralysis is typically associated with injury to the spinal cord. Immediate veterinary care is essential to diagnose and correct the problem. Proper transport of the dog is extremely important.

B.   Keep the dog quiet and restrict all activity.

C.   When you are moving your dog (as directed in D or E below), if the dog is in pain, you may wish to use a muzzle to prevent being bitten. Even a friendly dog may bite in reaction to pain.
However, use a muzzle only if the dog is not having difficulty breathing and has not been vomiting. If at any time the dog has difficulty breathing, remove the muzzle. Also, do not use a

muzzle if your dog has a flat face (e.g., a pug, boxer, English bulldog, etc.)

D. **If there is any chance your dog has damage to its spinal cord:**

(1) Obtain a plywood board to use as a stretcher. Slide the dog onto the board taking care to move the pet as little as possible. If the dog's back or neck is injured, improper movement could cause severe damage, including paralysis or death. If a board is not available, and you judge that the risk of delaying transport to a veterinarian outweighs the risk of moving the dog, try using a blanket or towel as a stretcher instead.

(2) Ideally, place the plywood board with the dog on it into your vehicle. If the board will not fit, slide the dog off of the board and onto the seat with as little movement of the pet as possible. If you have used a blanket or towel rather than a board, keep the blanket or towel under the dog when you put the pet into the car.

(3) Pack blankets around the dog to keep the pet warm. If you are concerned that the dog may slide off of the seat onto the floor, pack the floor area with a pillow or blankets. Place one or two 2-liter soda bottles filled with warm water (not hot water) against the dog. See illustrations on pages 125-126.

E. **If you are certain there is no damage to the spinal cord:**

(1) If the dog does not have any spinal-cord injury (i.e., has no problems with its neck or back) but is weak or paralyzed in its hind quarters, you can place a towel under the dog's abdomen for use as a sling to support the dog's weight. See the illustration on page 113.

(2) If the dog does not have any spinal-cord injury but is unable to support weight with either its front or back legs, you may lift and carry the dog to your car by placing one arm under the dog's neck and through the front legs and the other under the back third of the abdomen. Be careful not to make the back or neck arch. See illustration on page 25.

(3) Pack blankets around the dog to keep the pet warm. If you are concerned that the dog may slide off of the seat onto the floor, pack the floor area with a pillow or blankets. Place one or two 2-liter soda bottles filled with warm water (not hot water) against the dog. See illustrations on pages 125-126.

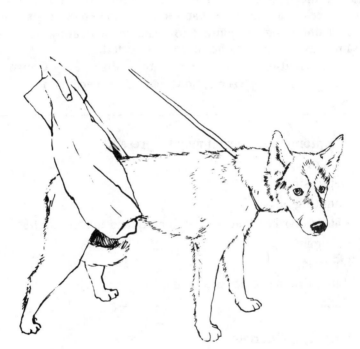

PROBLEM/CONDITION – PARVOVIRUS

Parvovirus is a highly contagious disease that is considered an emergency in dogs. Often dogs die within 24 hours after the onset of symptoms. The virus attacks the lining of the digestive tract causing severe vomiting and bloody diarrhea. The disease affects young, small and debilitated dogs most severely. Death is usually due to dehydration or overwhelming infection that spreads to the blood. Dogs that are infected with the virus can be contagious to other dogs for two weeks, and the virus can remain in the environment for years; proper disinfecting is required to ensure that healthy dogs entering the same environment do not become infected.

Vaccinations can prevent this disease. Consult your veterinarian regarding vaccinations and other precautions.

I. Symptoms (some or all may be present)

A. Loss of appetite

B. Depression

C. Vomiting

D. Watery diarrhea that is often bloody and usually foul-smelling

E. Pale gums

F. Shivering

G. Rapid decline in physical condition

H. Collapse

II. First-Aid Materials

A. Kaopectate®

B. Eyedropper or dosage syringe

C. Boiled hamburger and plain cooked rice

III. First Aid

A. Seek veterinary care immediately. Parvovirus is often fatal within 24 hours from the onset of symptoms.

B. While waiting for veterinary care, if there is no vomiting, feed the dog Kaopectate® using an eyedropper or dosage syringe:
   (1) 1 to 2 teaspoons for dogs weighing less than 20 pounds,
   (2) 3 to 4 teaspoons for dogs weighing 20 or more pounds.
C. If you are still delayed from receiving veterinary help, repeat Step B every 4 to 6 hours for adult dogs and every 2 to 4 hours for puppies less than 14 weeks old.
D. Withhold food for 2-4 hours if diarrhea is present and if there is no other symptom of illness. Withhold both food and water if the dog is also vomiting, but do not withhold water for more than 2 hours. Do not withhold water if the dog is not vomiting. The time period for withholding food should be based on whether your pet is a normal, healthy adult versus a puppy, an elderly dog or a dog with any special or compromising conditions. If your dog has diabetes or any other type of illness or medical condition, consult your veterinarian first before withholding food and water.
E. When you do resume feeding your dog, the best home remedy for diarrhea is to prepare a 50/50 mixture of boiled hamburger (drain off the water and fat) and plain cooked rice. Appropriate feedings are as follows:
   (1) 1/4 cup of the mixture 4 times per day for small dogs,
   (2) 1/2 cup of the mixture 4 times per day for medium dogs,
   (3) 3/4 cup of the mixture 4 times per day for large dogs.
   Your veterinarian may wish to adjust the servings or may recommend a prescription diet instead.
F. Note the frequency and substance of the diarrhea.
G. Parvovirus is often fatal, and professional veterinary care is critical for your dog's survival. The above procedures are appropriate while waiting for professional help, but they are not sufficient to save your dog.

PROBLEM/CONDITION – PENIS SHEATH DISCHARGE (BALANOPOSTHITIS)

Inflammation in the sheath surrounding the dog's penis (balanoposthitis) is common and is usually not cause for alarm, but the condition must be treated properly. It may be caused by foreign debris, a laceration, trauma or even a tumor. Dogs are prone to this type of inflammation and infection because there is a natural pocket or cavity in the sheath. When infection occurs, there is generally a cloudy discharge.

I. **Symptoms (one or both may be present)**
A. Cloudy, thick discharge from sheath
B. Dog licking sheath

II. **First-Aid Materials**
A. Antibiotic ointment (e.g., Polysporin®)

III. **First Aid**
A. Wipe discharge away from sheath.
B. Apply antibiotic ointment into sheath opening.
C. Seek veterinary care.

PROBLEM/CONDITION – PROTRUDING ORGANS

Various injuries and illnesses can result in the breakdown of vulnerable, weak areas of the dog's body. These areas include the eyes, abdomen and rectum. The things that most commonly protrude in a dog are a prolapsed rectum, an exposed prolapsed penis, a traumatic hernia with bowels exposed, and a popped-out eye. All of the above require immediate attention because these organs can dry out quickly causing permanent damage.

I. **Symptoms (one or both may be present)**

A. Most of these conditions can be recognized by observing the misplacement of the specific organ.

B. A prolapsed rectum may occur intermittently; the rectum may protrude only during times of straining, like during a bowel movement.

II. **First-Aid Materials**

A. Towel and/or gauze sponges

B. Contact-lens saline solution

C. Antibiotic ointment (e.g., Polysporin®)

III. **First Aid**

A. Contact a veterinarian immediately.

B. Soak a towel or gauze sponges with saline solution and apply to any area of protrusion. This will keep the organs from becoming dehydrated and increase the chances of a better prognosis. Also, by covering the protrusion, you will help prevent the dog from mutilating itself. With a disembowelment in particular, dogs will often chew on the exposed organs.

C. If the dog's eye is protruding, rinse the eye in saline every five minutes until a veterinarian can be reached. Do not apply pressure directly to the eye.

D. If the rectum is protruding, apply antibiotic ointment to help soothe the discomfort.

E. Use an Elizabethan collar if the dog is attempting to chew or scratch at the injury. See page 48.

PROBLEM/CONDITION – PROTRUDING PENIS (PARAPHIMOSIS)

Male dogs have a sheath that covers the penis. During mating or when the male dog is similarly aroused, the penis comes out from inside the sheath. Occasionally, hairs from the sheath get caught on the penis and prevent it from returning to the sheath. When this happens, the penis may swell, have its blood supply constricted by the sheath, and dry out.

I. Symptoms (some or all may be present)

A. Penis protruding from sheath

B. Swollen penis

C. Discolored (dark) penis

D. Dog licking genitals

II. First-Aid Materials

A. Contact-lens saline solution

B. Antibiotic ointment (e.g., Polysporin®)

C. Water-soluble lubricating jelly (e.g., K-Y™ Brand)

III. First Aid

A. Rinse penis with saline solution to remove any debris.

B. Apply antibiotic ointment to penis to prevent infection.

C. Apply water-soluble lubricating jelly to penis.

D. Gently remove any hairs that may be preventing retraction of the penis into the sheath, and then gently pull the sheath over the penis.

E. If the penis will not return to the sheath, immediate veterinary care is necessary to prevent the penis from drying out and dying.

If there is any delay is obtaining veterinary care, make sure that you reapply antibiotic ointment to the penis every 30 minutes. Apply an Elizabethan collar to prevent the dog from licking and chewing.

PROBLEM/CONDITION – RAT POISON

Rat poisons are laced in a grain base that intrigues dogs. When a dog eats rat poison, the poison interferes with the dog's ability to make vitamin K. Vitamin K is essential in causing blood to clot, and without the vitamin, a dog will hemorrhage internally. Because the symptoms from rat poison take several days to appear, early treatment is essential if an exposure is even suspected.

I.   Symptoms (some or all may be present)
A.   None for several days
B.   Weakness – frequently the first symptom
C.   Pale, white or bruised gums
D.   Bruises on the dog's body
E.   Bloody urine and/or stools
F.   Blue-green feces or vomitus – some rat baits contain a blue-green dye
G.   Death – may occur within 24 hours of first symptoms

II.   First-Aid Materials
A.   Hydrogen peroxide
B.   Eyedropper

III.   First Aid
A.   If exposure has occurred within 6 hours, immediately induce vomiting by feeding the dog 1 teaspoon of hydrogen peroxide (mixed with 1 teaspoon milk if available). If the dog will not drink the mixture or if no milk is available, then force-feed the dog the hydrogen peroxide using an eyedropper. If vomiting does not occur within 10 minutes, repeat the procedure twice.
B.   Regardless of whether you have been able to induce vomiting, seek veterinary care immediately. Your veterinarian will prescribe vitamin K as an antidote and may also prescribe medicines to slow absorption of the poison.

PROBLEM/CONDITION – SEIZURES

Seizures are common phenomena in dogs. They can be caused by a number of problems, including blood sugar imbalances (sometimes from diabetes), head trauma, various poisons or a buildup of wastes in the dog's circulation (as a result of organ failure). Some seizures may be hereditary in nature.

Seizures are one of the most frightening events to watch. Try hard to stay calm so that you are best able to tend to your dog's needs.

I. Symptoms (some or all may be present)

A. Confusion prior to the onset

B. Lack of awareness of its surroundings, including unresponsiveness to the owner

C. Distressed barking/crying

D. Loss of bladder and/or bowel control

E. Twitching or convulsing

F. Collapse

G. After the seizure has ended, the dog may be confused, uncoordinated and possibly blind for minutes or even hours.

II. First Aid

A. Note the time on a clock to measure the duration of the seizure.

B. If the seizure lasts more than 2 minutes, get veterinary help immediately; the condition may be life-threatening.

C. Move any objects that could cause the dog injury.

D. Block any stairways.

E. Never place your fingers in a dog's mouth during a seizure.

F. If the seizure stops and the dog appears lifeless, proceed as follows:

(1) Observe for breathing by watching the chest rise and fall.

(2) Establish an airway by removing any debris from the dog's mouth or by moving the tongue from the back of the throat. (See illustration page 42.) Check for breathing by watching the dog's chest rise and fall. **If the dog is breathing, proceed to Step G, and do not use CPR.**

(3) If the dog is still not breathing, lay the dog on its side (and throughout these procedures keep the dog on its side). Check for a pulse by placing a hand over the dog's chest just behind the shoulder blade (see page 44) to feel the heartbeat or by placing a hand in the groin area to feel the femoral pulse.

(4) **If the dog is still not breathing,**

    a) Cup your hand(s) over the dog's nose and mouth to form a seal. Deliver 1 breath into the pet every 2 seconds. If the seal is proper, you should observe the dog's chest rise and fall.

    b) If after you have delivered 5 breaths the dog does not show signs of breathing on its own or signs of consciousness, and there is no heartbeat, then have a helper place a hand just behind the dog's shoulder blades (as illustrated on page 44), and apply gentle but firm compressions downward (compressing 1/2 to 1 inch for a small dog up to 2 inches for a large dog) at a rate of 1 compression every 2 seconds. If a helper is not available, alternate delivering 2 breaths then 10 compressions. **Do not do any compressions if there is a pulse, no matter how faint.**

    c) Check for a pulse and breathing every 2 minutes. If there is no pulse and breathing, continue for up to 10 minutes before giving up.

G. If the seizure stops at home, even if the pet seems normal, consult your veterinarian as soon as possible.

PROBLEM/CONDITION –
SHOCK

Shock is an event that accompanies some diseases and injuries. It occurs when a series of compensatory mechanisms in the body goes awry. Problems that can cause shock include overwhelming infections, trauma (i.e., physical injury), severe vomiting and diarrhea, blood loss, and any other serious medical situation.

During the shock process, the body cannot keep up with the mixed signals that are being relayed. The body has a relative loss of blood due to changes in circulation or from bleeding. Changes in blood pressure shunt blood from vital organs like the heart, lungs, liver, kidneys and brain to other less important areas of the body. The result can be fatal if not treated early.

I.   **Symptoms (some or all may be present)**

A.   Note that immediately after an injury or other shock-inducing circumstance the symptoms of shock may be difficult to recognize, but they may develop quickly.

B.   The dog may be depressed and/or disoriented.

C.   The dog's vital signs may be decreased. Body temperature may fall, breathing may be shallow and pulse may be weak.

D.   The dog's feet, tail, and ears may feel cold to the touch.

II. **First-Aid Materials**

A.   2-liter soda bottle

B.   Blanket or towels

C.   Thermometer

III. **First Aid**

A.   Shock is a danger in virtually all medical emergencies. You should treat your dog for shock following any serious trauma regardless of whether you observe any symptoms.

B.   Keep the dog warm by placing a 2-liter soda bottle filled with warm water (not hot water) against the dog. See illustration below. Cover the dog with a towel or blanket.

C.   Monitor the dog's vital signs (temperature, pulse and respirations) every 15 minutes and record the information. Try to keep the dog's temperature within the range of 100-102.5 degrees Fahrenheit. If the dog's temperature rises above 102.5 degrees Fahrenheit, remove the warm soda bottle. If the dog's temperature falls below 100 degrees, place an additional warm-water soda bottle against the dog, but make sure the water is not hot and make sure the bottle is against the dog and not on top of or underneath the dog. See illustration on page 126.

D.   Contact a veterinarian immediately so that anti-shock drugs, and possibly intravenous fluids, can be administered.

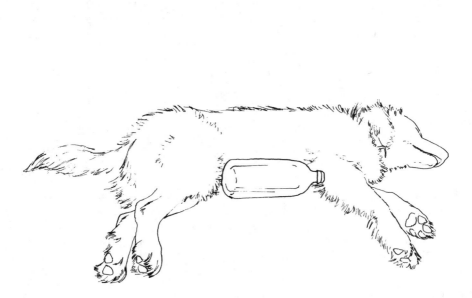

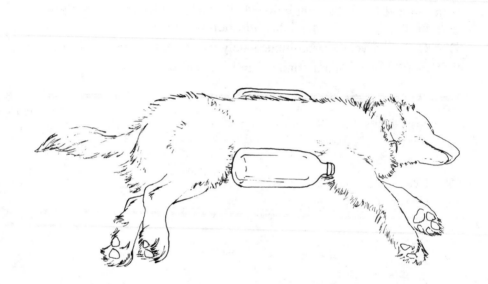

PROBLEM/CONDITION – SLIPPED (HERNIATED) DISC DISEASE

Disc disease in dogs causes a variety of symptoms depending on the location and severity of the condition. Symptoms may range from mild neck or back pain to extreme pain or paralysis. When a disc slips out of place, it applies pressure to the spinal cord, or nerves leading from the cord, creating the pain or paralysis. Mild cases may quickly worsen; prompt veterinary care is urgent.

I. Symptoms (some or all may be present)

A. Back or neck pain

B. Reluctance to move or participate in routine activities

C. Hesitation to climb or jump

D. Crying when petted or lifted

E. Difficulty lifting head

F. Difficulty eating

G. Lameness

H. Folding under or dragging toes or back legs

I. Hunched appearance when walking

J. Pain during bowel movements

K. Paralysis

II. First-Aid Materials

A. Muzzle

B. Blanket or plywood board (cut to fit your dog and your car)

III. First Aid

A. Keep the dog quiet and restrict all activity. See a veterinarian as soon as possible.

B. When you are moving your dog (as directed in C below), if the dog is in pain, you may wish to use a muzzle to prevent being bitten. Even a friendly dog may bite in reaction to pain. However, use a muzzle only if the dog is not having difficulty breathing and has not been vomiting. If at any time the dog has difficulty breathing, remove the muzzle. Also, do not use a muzzle if your dog has a flat face (e.g., a pug, boxer, English bulldog, etc.).

C.   If your dog is unable to walk, obtain a plywood board to use as a stretcher. Slide the dog onto the board taking care to move the pet as little as possible. Improper movement could cause severe damage, including paralysis or death.

D.   Ideally, place the plywood board with the dog on it into your vehicle. If the board will not fit, slide the dog off of the board and onto the seat with as little movement of the pet as possible.

E.   Pack blankets around the dog to keep the pet warm. If you are concerned that the dog may slide off of the seat onto the floor, pack the floor area with a pillow or blankets. Place one or two 2-liter soda bottles filled with warm water (not hot water) against the dog. See illustrations on pages 125-126.

PROBLEM/CONDITION – SMOKE INHALATION

Smoke inhalation is often the cause of death when a dog is trapped in a fire. Smoke damages the respiratory tract thereby interfering with normal breathing; in addition, smoke contains the deadly gas carbon monoxide. It is important to note that the symptoms of smoke inhalation might not appear for as long as 1 to 2 days after the exposure.

I. **Symptoms (some or all may be present)**

A. Difficult breathing – short, shallow or rapid breaths, panting or coughing

B. Purple, blue or pale gums and tongue

C. Disorientation

D. Coma

E. Death

II. **First Aid Materials**

A. 2-liter soda bottle

III. **First Aid**

A. Move the dog away from the smoke.

B. Check for breathing. You should be able to see the dog's chest rise and fall.

C. If the dog is not breathing, establish an airway by removing any debris from the dog's mouth or by moving the tongue from the back of the throat. (See illustration page 42.) Check for breathing by watching the dog's chest rise and fall. **If the dog is breathing, proceed to Step E, and do not use CPR.**

D. **If the dog is not breathing,**

　(1) Lay the dog on its side (and throughout Step D keep the dog on its side). Check for a pulse by placing a hand over

the dog's chest just behind the shoulder blade (see page 44) to feel the heartbeat or by placing a hand in the groin area to feel the femoral pulse.

(2) Cup your hand(s) over the dog's nose and mouth to form a seal. Deliver 1 breath into the pet every 2 seconds. If the seal is proper, you should observe the dog's chest rise and fall.

(3) If after you have delivered 5 breaths the dog does not show signs of breathing on its own or signs of consciousness, and there is no heartbeat, then have a helper place a hand just behind the dog's shoulder blades (as illustrated on page 43), and apply gentle but firm compressions downward (compressing 1/2 to 1 inch for a small dog up to 2 inches for a large dog) at a rate of 1 compression every 2 seconds. If a helper is not available, alternate delivering 2 breaths then 10 compressions. **Do not do any compressions if there is a pulse, no matter how faint.**

(4) Check for a pulse and breathing every 2 minutes. If there is no pulse and breathing, continue for up to 10 minutes before giving up.

E. Avoid all stress. The least amount of stress may precipitate a crisis when the dog is having difficulty breathing.

F. Do not monitor vital signs.

G. Plan the handling of the dog to minimize excitement. Never hold the dog tightly.

H. Keep the dog in an upright position (i.e., belly down). Never lay the dog on its back or side because those positions make breathing more difficult by putting extra pressure on the chest.

I. Fill a 2-liter soda bottle with warm (not hot) water and place it against the dog. See illustration on page 125.

J. Contact a veterinarian immediately. It is easy to underestimate the severity of the dog's condition because some symptoms might not appear until 12 to 48 hours after smoke inhalation occurs.

PROBLEM/CONDITION – SNAIL BAIT

Snail bait is poisonous to pets because it contains the chemical metaldehyde. This product, like rat poison, is made with a tasty base that attracts not only snails but also dogs.

I. Symptoms (some or all may be present)

A. Loss of coordination

B. Muscle tremors or convulsions

C. Increased heart rate

II. First-Aid Materials

A. Hydrogen peroxide

B. Eyedropper or dosage syringe

III. First Aid

A. Induce vomiting early if exposure is suspected. Do not attempt to induce vomiting if the pet is showing signs of poisoning (i.e., if it appears uncoordinated or is having muscle tremors or convulsions) because the pet could aspirate vomit into its lungs. To induce vomiting, feed the dog 1 teaspoon of hydrogen peroxide (mixed with 1 teaspoon milk if available). If the dog will not drink the mixture or if there is no milk available, then force-feed the dog the hydrogen peroxide using an eyedropper or dosage syringe. If vomiting does not occur within 10 minutes, repeat the procedure twice.

B. Contact a veterinarian immediately.

PROBLEM/CONDITION – SNAKE BITES

Bites from poisonous snakes pose a threat in many areas of the country. The severity of the bite will depend upon the type of snake, the age of the dog, the size of the dog, the number of bites, the location of the bites, and the amount of venom injected. Unless you are skilled at identifying snakes and witness the attack first-hand, it may be difficult to determine whether the snake is poisonous. Therefore, it is urgent that you seek veterinary care immediately. If you wait for obvious symptoms to develop, your veterinarian might be too late to save your pet.

I. **Symptoms (some or all may be present)**
A. Poisonous snake bites often appear as two punctures on the skin.
B. Nonpoisonous snake bites are often shaped like a "U" because nonpoisonous snakes tend to have many teeth.
C. Poisonous snake bites tend to be especially painful.
D. The area around a poisonous snake bite will swell and may show bruising.
E. The dog may become depressed, paralyzed, comatose, and may die. These symptoms may be preceded by respiratory distress or by digestive upset.

II. **First-Aid Materials**
A. 2-liter soda bottle
B. Antibiotic ointment (e.g., Polysporin®)

III. **First Aid**
A. If you suspect that the bite is from a poisonous snake (see the symptoms listed above),
    (1) Restrict activity, and keep the dog calm.
    (2) Keep the dog warm by placing 2-liter soda bottles filled with

warm water (not hot water) against the pet. (See illustrations on pages 125-126.)

(3) Rush the dog to a veterinarian.

B. If you suspect that the bite is from a nonpoisonous snake,

(1) Wash the bite wound with soap and water, and then apply antibiotic ointment.

(2) Seek veterinary care immediately. The bite could be from a poisonous snake, and even if it is not, your dog may need antibiotic therapy because reptiles have many infectious bacteria in their mouths.

PROBLEM/CONDITION – SPIDER BITES, ANT BITES AND SCORPION STINGS

Several varieties of spiders, ants and scorpions can cause injury and illness in dogs. The brown recluse spider and black widow spider are particularly venomous, though fortunately they are much less common than other spiders. Most ants are harmless in small numbers, but a colony of ants can pose a real risk. Scorpions are not native to much of the United States, but they (and tarantulas) are sometimes sold in pet stores.

It should be noted that some symptoms from spiders, ants and scorpions may not appear until 3 or 4 days after the bites or sting. These delayed symptoms may include paleness, blood in urine, fever, vomiting and shock.

I. **Symptoms (some or all may be present)**

A. Salivation, if bite or sting is in the dog's mouth

B. Irritated area on skin

C. Open sore on body

D. Painful area

E. Muscle pain

F. Muscle contractions

G. Fever

H. Rapid or difficult breathing

I. Paleness

J. Vomiting

K. Blood in urine

L. Shock

M. Paralysis

N. Death

II. First-Aid Materials

A. Ice

B. Towel

III. First Aid

A. Seek veterinary care immediately.

B. Wrap some ice in a cloth and place it against the wound. (The ice will slow the spread of venom.) Apply the wrapped ice over the swollen, painful areas for 10 minutes. Wait 5 minutes, and then reapply for another 10 minutes.

C. If possible, identify the spider, ants or scorpion (to aid in proper veterinary care).

PROBLEM/CONDITION – STRYCHNINE POISONING

Strychnine is sometimes an ingredient in products sold to kill insects and rodents. The products are laced with a sweetener to attract the animal and generally contain enough strychnine that even ingestion of a small amount of the product will kill the pest. Unfortunately, strychnine is highly poisonous, and even a small amount will likely kill your dog. If your dog does ingest strychnine, immediate action is necessary.

I. Symptoms (some or all may be present)

A. Symptoms may appear within 2 hours of ingestion.

B. The dog may appear to be apprehensive or nervous.

C. Stiffness may develop, leading to severe seizures. These seizures can be provoked or exacerbated by stimulus (e.g., a loud noise).

D. Exhaustion and death may shortly follow the onset of symptoms.

II. First-Aid Materials

A. Hydrogen peroxide

B. Eyedropper or dosage syringe

III. First Aid

A. Induce vomiting if the pet is conscious and there has been a suspected exposure. To induce vomiting, feed the dog 1 teaspoon of hydrogen peroxide (mixed with 1 teaspoon milk if available). If the dog will not drink the mixture or if there is no milk available, then force-feed the dog the hydrogen peroxide using an eyedropper or dosage syringe. If vomiting does not occur within 10 minutes, repeat the procedure twice.

B. Keep your dog from injuring itself during any seizures by blocking off stairways and moving furnishings. If seizures do occur, follow the instructions on treatment for seizures, page 122.

C. Keep the dog in a calm, quiet environment.

D. Immediately seek veterinary help.

PROBLEM/CONDITION – TIGHT COLLAR

If your dog is still growing or is gaining weight, its collar may become too tight. The collar could cause difficulty breathing and it could actually cut into the skin.

I.   Symptoms (some or all may be present)

A.   Dog scratching/pawing at its neck

B.   Difficulty breathing

C.   Bloody discharge or putrid smell from collar area

II.   First-Aid Materials

A.   Antibiotic ointment (e.g., Polysporin®)

B.   Scissors

III. First Aid

A.   If the collar has not grown into the skin, simply loosen it or remove it.

B.   If the collar has grown into the skin:

   (1) Clip hair away from the collar.

   (2) Try to find a place where you can gently slip the scissors under the collar to cut it off. If you cannot get the scissors under the collar, seek veterinary assistance to have the collar removed.

   (3) Apply antibiotic ointment to the wound.

   (4) Seek veterinary care to treat for possible infection.

PROBLEM/CONDITION – TOAD POISONING

     Many toads produce venom from glands in their skin. The amount of venom and its potency varies depending on the type of toad. The severity of symptoms you can expect your dog to exhibit from toad poisoning will depend upon the amount of exposure as well as the strength of the venom.

I.   Symptoms (some or all may be present)
A. Salivation
B. Rubbing mouth
C. Shaking head
D. Dry heaves
E. Vomiting
F. Weakness
G. Difficulty breathing
H. Blue gums
I. Seizures
J. Collapse
K. Death

II. First-Aid Materials
A. Fresh water
B. Eyedropper or dosage syringe

III. First Aid
A. Using an eyedropper or dosage syringe, flush the dog's mouth with fresh water to remove excess venom.
B. If possible, identify the type of toad.
C. Seek veterinary care.

PROBLEM/CONDITION – TORN TOENAIL

It is important to keep your dog's toenails trimmed to prevent them from catching on carpets and outdoor hazards. If your dog does tear a toenail, it may be painful for the pet, but the nail will eventually grow back.

I. Symptoms (some or all may be present)

A. Lameness

B. Nail hanging from paw

C. Blood coming from nail bed

D. Dog shaking its paw

II. First-Aid Materials

A. Muzzle

B. Nonstick bandages and gauze wrap

C. Tape

D. Nail trimmers

III. First Aid

A. Apply a muzzle if there is no evidence of difficulty breathing or nausea. If at any time the dog has difficulty breathing, remove the muzzle. Also, do not use a muzzle if your dog has a flat face (e.g., a pug, boxer, English bulldog, etc.).

B. Do not attempt to remove a dangling nail. (You may, however, trim the nail to help prevent further injury to the nail bed.) If the paw is bleeding, apply gentle but firm pressure to the paw to stop the bleeding.

C. If the bleeding persists, wrap the foot using a nonstick bandage, gauze wrap and tape. (See Wrapping a Wound on page 37.)

D. See a veterinarian to have the nail trimmed or removed and for treatment to prevent infection.

E. Keep the dog's healthy toenails trimmed to prevent injuries in the future.

PROBLEM/CONDITION – URINARY-TRACT IRRITATIONS

Urinary-tract problems are common in dogs of all ages and breeds. Urinary-tract irritations may be caused by a variety of problems including infections and bladder or kidney stones. These problems can quickly develop into emergencies because of the amount of distress the dog experiences. In the worst case scenario, a dog may be unable to urinate because of a blockage; the poisons normally excreted in the urine accumulate in the dog's system causing severe illness which may include permanent organ damage, coma and death. If urinary-tract blockage is left untreated, death is imminent.

I.   Symptoms (some or all may be present)

A.   Broken house habits (i.e., urinating in the house)

B.   Urinating more frequently

C.   Straining while trying to urinate

D.   Crying while urinating

E.   Blood in the urine

F.   Inability to urinate

G.   Other generalized signs of illness (i.e., changes in behavior)

II.   First-Aid Materials

A.   2-liter soda bottle

III. First Aid

A.   Observe the dog for urine output. The dog should be able to excrete at least small amounts of urine.

B.   If no urine production is detected, the situation is urgent; the dog's urinary system may be blocked, and blockage is life-threatening. A veterinarian should be contacted immediately.

C.   Monitor the dog's vital signs until a veterinarian can be reached.

D.   Keep the dog warm by placing a 2-liter soda bottle filled with warm water (not hot water) against the dog.

E.   Avoid lifting the dog around its abdomen to prevent discomfort and possible rupture of the bladder.

F.   Even if urine is being produced, consult a veterinarian as soon as possible for diagnosis and treatment before the situation turns into a life-threatening blockage.

G.   Do not encourage the dog to eat or drink if you suspect there is a blockage because your veterinarian may determine that a urinary catheter is necessary, and insertion of the catheter may require a general anesthetic.

PROBLEM/CONDITION – UTERUS INFECTION

Infection of the uterus can occur for no apparent reason in a seemingly normal, healthy canine. The cause is generally hormonal, and prior to symptoms, there is no method of predicting when or whether it might occur. Infections of the uterus can be fatal. The unspayed, older adult female is at highest risk. When a dog's uterus becomes infected, it can fill with pus. Eventually the organ can burst, spilling infection into the abdomen, or the infection might be absorbed from the uterus into the bloodstream.

I. Symptoms (some or all may be present)

A. Increased thirst that precedes other signs

B. General signs of illness such as loss of appetite, vomiting, diarrhea or depression

C. A cloudy, foul-smelling discharge coming from the vulvar area under the tail

D. Tense and distended abdomen

II. First-Aid Materials

A. 2-liter soda bottle

III. First Aid

A. If any of these symptoms are noted, contact a veterinarian immediately. The dog may require an emergency spay before the uterus ruptures.

B. Do not lift the dog by putting extra pressure on the abdomen; lifting in that manner may cause the uterus to rupture.

C. To help prevent shock, place a 2-liter soda bottle filled with warm water (not hot water) next to the dog (as illustrated on page 125).

PROBLEM/CONDITION – VOMITING

The goal in helping a dog that is vomiting is to comfort the pet and lessen the symptoms until the cause can be determined. There are many causes of vomiting including dietary changes, infections, poisons, and obstruction from foreign objects that are undigestible. Sometimes vomiting is accompanied by diarrhea.

I. Symptoms (some or all may be present)
A. Loss of appetite
B. Salivation
C. Retching
D. Vomiting
E. Painful abdomen

II. First-Aid Materials
A. Boiled hamburger and plain cooked rice

III. First Aid
A. If the dog is vomiting, withhold food and water for 2-4 hours. (But if your dog has diabetes or any other type of illness or medical condition, consult your veterinarian first before withholding food and water.) Do not withhold food and water from a puppy or elderly dog for more than 2 hours. If symptoms persist, worsen or return within this 2-4 hour period, contact your veterinarian.
B. Note the frequency and substance of the vomiting. Is the food undigested or is the vomitus watery?
C. Note how long after a meal the vomiting occurred.
D. When you do resume feeding your dog, prepare a 50/50 mixture of boiled hamburger (drain off the water and fat) and plain cooked rice. Appropriate feedings are as follows:

(1) 1/4 cup of the mixture 4 times per day for small dogs,

(2) 1/2 cup of the mixture 4 times per day for medium dogs,

(3) 3/4 cup of the mixture 4 times per day for large dogs.

Your veterinarian may wish to adjust the servings or may recommend a prescription diet instead.

E.   Resume normal feeding within 2 days.

PROBLEM/CONDITION – YARD CHEMICALS

A variety of chemicals in fertilizers and pesticides can cause illness either from inhalation, contact or ingestion. Symptoms of illness may be delayed for days, but may be quite severe. Avoid exposing your dog to these toxins by keeping your dog off the treated area during the yard fertilization or spraying and for at least 48 hours afterward (or more if the chemical manufacturer advises a longer period of time). If you are using an insecticide indoors, keep your dog out of the room until the chemicals have dissipated. Never spray your dog with an insecticide that is not labeled specifically for use on dogs.

I. Symptoms (some or all may be present)
A. Listlessness
B. Loss of appetite
C. Difficulty breathing
D. Salivation
E. Vomiting
F. Diarrhea
G. Skin irritation from contact (typically the pads of the feet)

II. First Aid Materials
A. Shampoo

III. First Aid
A. If the dog gets chemicals on its fur, bathe the dog with dog shampoo (or any mild moisturizing shampoo if dog shampoo is not available). While restraining the dog, apply the shampoo and let it stand for 10 minutes before rinsing well.
B. Seek veterinary assistance for additional advice and treatment.

SYMPTOM – BLEEDING
(from abrasions and lacerations)

The most common problems that cause bleeding include abrasions and lacerations. When external bleeding does occur, you must get it under control as quickly as possible. An injury that causes significant blood loss may cause the dog to go into shock.

I. **First-Aid Materials**

A. Clean towel

B. Gauze sponges

C. Nonstick adhesive tape

D. Nonstick bandages

E. Gauze wrap

F. Antibiotic ointment (e.g., Polysporin®)

II. **First Aid**

A. Using a clean towel or sterile sponges, apply direct pressure to the area of bleeding for 5-10 minutes. If the bleeding does not stop, you may apply a wrap using the following procedure:

(1) Press nonstick bandage to wound.

(2) Secure nonstick bandage to wound by wrapping gauze around the dog's leg or body. The gauze should be pulled snug but not tight. The wrap should not restrict the dog's circulation or breathing.

(3) Secure the gauze by applying adhesive tape to the wrap.

(4) Monitor the pet for any evidence of swelling to the limb below the wrap. If swelling occurs, the wrap is too tight, and you should loosen it immediately. If the dog's breathing is hindered, also loosen or remove the wrap.

(5) Do not attempt to apply a tourniquet, even if the injury is a

severed tail.

B. If the bleeding was difficult to stop, do not attempt to clean the wound or apply antibiotic ointment because the clot may be disrupted and severe hemorrhage may resume.

C. For future reference, note the amount of blood loss from the injury.

D. For serious lacerations, confine the dog to prevent activity.

E. For minor wounds, apply antibiotic ointment.

F. If the injury seems severe, treat the dog for shock as follows:

(1) Keep the dog warm by placing a 2-liter soda bottle filled with warm water (not hot water) against the dog. Cover the dog with a towel or blanket.

(2) Monitor the dog's vital signs (temperature, pulse and respirations) every 15 minutes and record the information. Try to keep the dog's temperature within the range of 100 to 103 degrees Fahrenheit. If the dog's temperature rises above 103 degrees Fahrenheit, remove the warm soda bottle. If the dog's temperature falls below 100 degrees, place an additional warm-water soda bottle against the dog, but make sure the water is not hot and make sure the bottle is against the dog and not on top of or underneath the dog.

G. Call your veterinarian immediately. For best healing, lacerations should be repaired as soon as possible (ideally within one hour after the injury). As more time elapses, the wound becomes contaminated and may not be able to be closed.

SYMPTOM –
BLEEDING
(from bite wound abscesses)

Sometimes minor wounds can become infected, especially if the cause of the wound is a bite. With bite wounds, the skin may heal with an infection beneath it. The dog's immune system will attempt to isolate the infection, and the result can be the formation of a pocket of bacteria and pus called an abscess. The abscess may spread either inward through the bloodstream or outward through the skin. If the infection spreads inward, the resulting infection can damage internal organs. If it moves outward, it may rupture, and blood and pus will drain from the opening. The opening will appear as if something has eaten a hole in the animal, and it may be as large as a half-inch or more in diameter. The rupture and accompanying drainage may look frightening, but it is actually good for the dog because it helps get rid of the infection.

I. **First-Aid Materials**

A. Warm compresses

B. Paper towels

C. Antibiotic ointment (e.g., Polysporin®)

II. **First Aid**

A. Locate wound. (Look for healed puncture wounds.)

B. Take pet's temperature.

C. Apply warm compresses to area to promote drainage of the abscess until a veterinarian can be contacted. The warm compresses may cause the abscess to rupture and spill out blood and pus. This will make the pet feel better because the infection is being removed from the body. Be prepared to clean up a mess.

D. Apply antibiotic ointment to the wound.

E. Contact a veterinarian. Your pet may need prescription antibiotics or may require sedation to promote better drainage of an infected wound.

SYMPTOM – BLEEDING
(from gunshot wounds)

If your dog is ever a victim of a shooting, it may be critical that you get the bleeding under control as fast as possible. Also, you may need to treat the dog for shock. (See Problem/Condition - Shock.)

I.   First-Aid Materials

A.   Clean towel

B.   Gauze sponges

C.   Nonstick adhesive tape

D.   Nonstick bandages

E.   Gauze wrap

II.   First Aid

A.   Locate the source of bleeding.

B.   DO NOT attempt to remove pellets or bullets.

C.   Using a clean towel or sterile sponges, apply direct pressure to the area of bleeding for 5-10 minutes. If the bleeding does not stop, you may apply a wrap using the following procedure:

(1)   Press nonstick bandage to wound.

(2)   Secure nonstick bandage to wound by wrapping gauze around the dog's leg or body. The gauze should be pulled snug but not tight. The wrap should not restrict the dog's circulation or breathing.

(3)   Secure the gauze by applying adhesive tape to the wrap.

(4)   Monitor the pet for any evidence of swelling to the limb below the wrap. If swelling occurs, then the wrap is too tight, and you should loosen it immediately. If the dog's

breathing is hindered, also loosen or remove the wrap.

D. For future reference, note the amount of blood loss from the injury.

E. If the bleeding was difficult to stop, do not attempt to clean the wound or apply antibiotic ointment because the clot may be disrupted and severe hemorrhage may resume.

F. Confine the dog to prevent activity.

G. Treat the dog for shock as follows:

(1) Keep the dog warm by placing a 2-liter soda bottle filled with warm water (not hot water) against the dog. Cover the dog with a towel or blanket.

(2) Monitor the dog's vital signs (temperature, pulse and respirations) every 15 minutes and record the information. Try to keep the dog's temperature within the range of 100 to 103 degrees Fahrenheit. If the dog's temperature rises rises above 103 degrees Fahrenheit, remove the warm soda bottle. If the dog's temperature falls below 100 degrees, place an additional warm-water soda bottle against the dog, but make sure the water is not hot and make sure the bottle is against the dog and not on top of or underneath the dog.

H. Call your veterinarian immediately.

SYMPTOM –
BLEEDING
(external and internal from trauma, in general)

Often an emergency will involve some type of hemorrhage. The bleeding may be mild, moderate, or severe. Severe hemorrhage may involve the severing of an artery, injury to a large muscle mass, a fracture of a bone, toxicity due to rat poisoning, a ruptured tumor, or internal trauma to an organ. If the blood pools quickly or pumps in spurts, you can assume it is serious. Immediate action is required to prevent shock.

Whenever there is serious trauma, there is a possibility of internal bleeding and shock. Seek veterinary assistance immediately.

I.   First-Aid Materials
A.   Clean towel
B.   Gauze sponges
C.   Nonstick adhesive tape
D.   Nonstick bandages
E.   Gauze wrap

II.   First Aid
A.   Locate the source of bleeding.
B.   Using a clean towel or gauze sponges, apply direct pressure to the wound for 5-10 minutes.
C.   A wrap may be applied to the wound if bleeding does not stop:
   (1)   Press nonstick bandages to wound.
   (2)   Secure nonstick bandages to wound by wrapping gauze around the dog's leg or body. The gauze should be pulled snug but not tight. The wrap should not restrict the dog's

circulation or breathing.

(3) Secure the gauze by applying adhesive tape to the wrap.

(4) Monitor the pet for any evidence of swelling to the limb below the wrap. If swelling occurs, then the wrap is too tight, and you should loosen it immediately. If the dog's breathing is hindered, also loosen or remove the wrap.

D. If the bleeding has stopped, do not attempt to clean the wound or apply antibiotic ointment because the clot may be disrupted and severe hemorrhage may resume.

E. For future reference, note the amount of blood loss from the injury.

F. Treat the dog for shock as follows:

(1) Keep the dog warm by placing a 2-liter soda bottle filled with warm water (not hot water) against the dog. Cover the dog with a towel or blanket.

(2) Monitor the dog's vital signs (temperature, pulse and respirations) every 15 minutes and record the information. Try to keep the dog's temperature within the range of 100 to 103 degrees Fahrenheit. If the dog's temperature rises above 103 degrees Fahrenheit, remove the warm soda bottle. If the dog's temperature falls below 100 degrees, place an additional warm-water soda bottle against the dog, but make sure the water is not hot and make sure the bottle is against the dog and not on top of or underneath the dog.

G. Lacerations are best repaired within a 1-hour time frame. As time elapses, the wound becomes contaminated and may not be able to be closed.

H. Trauma may be accompanied by internal bleeding. (Symptoms include pale gums, weakness, bruising on the skin or gums, distended abdomen and/or difficulty breathing.) After any severe trauma, make sure your pet receives veterinary care to identify any problems you may be unable to detect.

SYMPTOM – BREATHING DIFFICULTIES

I.   Problems/Conditions with that Symptom

A.   Heart disease

B.   Lung disease

C.   Heat stroke

D.   Internal bleeding

E.   Shock/trauma

F.   Anemia

G.   Fractured ribs

H.   Poisoning

I.   Asthma

J.   Obstruction of the airway

K.   Bee and scorpion stings

L.   Smoke inhalation

M.   Most other medical emergencies

II.   First-Aid Materials

A.   Two 2-liter soda bottles

B.   Blanket

III.   First Aid

A.   Avoid all stress. The least bit of stress may precipitate a crisis when the pet cannot breathe.

B.   Do not monitor vital signs.

C.   Plan the handling of the dog to minimize excitement. Never hold tightly.

D.   Never lay the dog on its back or side because this will compromise oxygen exchange by putting extra pressure on the chest.

E.   Contact a veterinarian immediately.

SYMPTOM –
BUMPS/LUMPS

I. Problems/Conditions with that Symptom

A. Allergy/hives

B. Insect bites and stings

C. Drug reactions

D. Bite wounds

E. Tumor, cyst or swollen lymph nodes

II. First-Aid Materials

A. Towel(s)

B. Ice

C. Benedryl® or diphenhydramine elixir (12.5 mg/ml liquid)

III. First Aid

A. If the dog is uncomfortable, place a towel moistened with cold water, or ice wrapped in a towel, over the irritated areas. This is especially soothing for hives and insect bites and stings.

B. If you are unable to reach a veterinarian, and you suspect that the bumps/lumps are hives, allergies, insect bites or insect stings, you may give the dog Benedryl® or diphenhydramine elixir (12.5 mg/ml liquid) as follows:

(1) 1/8 teaspoon for dogs weighing less than five pounds.

(2) 1/4 teaspoon for dogs weighing 5 to 20 pounds.

(3) 1/2 teaspoon for dogs weighing 21 to 60 pounds.

(4) 1 teaspoon for dogs weighing more than 60 pounds.

C. Seek veterinary help. There are medications that may help give relief.

SYMPTOM –
CHOKING

I. Problems/Conditions with that Symptom
A. Foreign body
B. Aspiration of fluid
C. Nausea

II. First-Aid Materials
A. 1-inch roll of tape
B. Pencil with eraser

III. First Aid
A. Open the dog's mouth to see whether a foreign object is lodged in the dog's mouth or throat, but take care to prevent being bitten. If necessary, use a small roll of first-aid tape as a wedge to keep the dog's mouth open to allow better access and to protect you from the dog's teeth. (See illustration on page 76.)
B. If the dog's airway is not blocked, wait for veterinary assistance before attempting to remove any object; your efforts could do more harm than good. If the airway is blocked, use the eraser end of a pencil to try gently to dislodge the object.
C. If fluid is causing the choking, try wiping the fluid from the mouth using a tissue. You may need to hold the dog with its head lower than its chest for approximately 5 to 10 seconds in order for the fluid to drain. Repeat this process no more than five times.
D. If the pet becomes unconscious:
    (1) Observe for breathing by watching the dog's chest rise and fall.
    (2) **If the dog is breathing,** proceed to Step F; do not use CPR.
E. **If the dog is not breathing,** proceed with CPR as follows:

(1) Establish an airway by removing any debris from the dog's mouth or by moving the tongue from the back of the throat. (See illustration page 42.) Check for breathing by watching the dog's chest rise and fall. If the dog is breathing, proceed to Step F; do not use CPR.

(2) If the dog is not breathing, lay the dog on its side (and throughout these procedures keep the dog on its side). Check for a pulse by placing a hand over the dog's chest just behind the shoulder blade (see page 44) to feel the heartbeat or by placing a hand in the groin area to feel the femoral pulse.

(3) Cup your hand(s) over the dog's nose and mouth to form a seal. Deliver 1 breath into the pet every 2 seconds. If the seal is proper, you should observe the dog's chest rise and fall.

(4) If after you have delivered 5 breaths the dog does not show signs of breathing on its own or signs of consciousness, and there is no heartbeat, then have a helper place a hand just behind the dog's shoulder blades (as illustrated on page 44), and apply gentle but firm compressions downward (compressing 1/2 to 1 inch for a small dog up to as much as 2 inches for a large dog) at a rate of 1 compression every 2 seconds. If a helper is not available, alternate delivering 2 breaths then 10 compressions. **Do not do any compressions if there is a pulse, no matter how faint.**

(5) Check for a pulse and breathing every 2 minutes. If there is no pulse and breathing, continue for up to 10 minutes before giving up.

F. Sedation may be necessary to remove a foreign object; if your attempt at home is unsuccessful, seek immediate veterinary care.

G. Regardless of whether the object has been removed, have your dog checked by a veterinarian as soon as possible for lacerations in the mouth and throat.

SYMPTOM – COLLAPSE

I. Problems/Conditions with that Symptom

A. Anemia

B. Bloat (gastric dilation volvulus) or twisted stomach

C. Diabetes

D. Heart disease

E. Heat stroke

F. Hypothermia

G. Infections

H. Internal bleeding

I. Lung disease

J. Poisonings

K. Seizures

L. Shock/trauma

M. Urinary blockage

II. First-Aid Materials

A. Two 2-liter soda bottles

B. Blanket

C. Honey or Karo® syrup (if collapse is from diabetes)

III. First Aid

A. If the dog is diabetic, the cause of the collapse could be insulin shock. If so, rub the dog's gums with honey or Karo® syrup.

B. If the pet is unconscious, check for breathing by watching the dog's chest rise and fall.

C. **If the dog is breathing,** proceed to Step E. Do not use CPR.

D. **If the dog is not breathing,**

    (1) Establish an airway by removing any debris from the dog's

mouth or by moving the tongue from the back of the throat. (See illustration page 42.) Check for breathing by watching the dog's chest rise and fall. If the dog is breathing, proceed to Step E, and do not use CPR.

(2) If the dog is not breathing, lay the dog on its side (and throughout these procedures keep the dog on its side). Check for a pulse by placing a hand over the dog's chest just behind the shoulder blade (see page 44) or by placing a hand in the groin area to feel the femoral pulse.

(3) Cup your hand(s) over the dog's nose and mouth to form a seal. Deliver 1 breath into the pet every 2 seconds. If the seal is proper, you should see the dog's chest rise and fall.

(4) If after you have delivered 5 breaths the dog does not show signs of breathing on its own or signs of consciousness, and there is no heartbeat, then have a helper place a hand just behind the dog's shoulder blades (as illustrated on page 44), and apply gentle but firm compressions downward (compressing 1/2 to 1 inch for a small dog up to as much as 2 inches for a large dog) at a rate of 1 compression every 2 seconds. If a helper is not available, alternate delivering 2 breaths then 10 compressions. **Do not do any compressions if there is a pulse, no matter how faint.**

(5) Check for a pulse and breathing every 2 minutes. If there is no pulse and breathing, continue for up to 10 minutes before giving up.

E. If the dog is conscious, proceed as follows:

(1) Keep the pet calm, and avoid unnecessary stress. Do not monitor vital signs, and do not use excessive restraint or cause excessive movement. Plan the handling of the dog to minimize stress. Never hold the dog tightly.

(2) Lay the dog upright (i.e., belly down). (If the dog is on its back or side, there is extra pressure on the chest making it harder for the pet to breathe.)

F. Seek immediate veterinary care.

SYMPTOM –
COUGHING

I.   **Problems/Conditions with that Symptom**
A.   Heart disease
B.   Lung disease
C.   Infections
D.   Bronchitis or tonsillitis
E.   Asthma
F.   Smoke inhalation
G.   Obstruction from a foreign object

II. **First-Aid Materials**
A.   Chicken bouillon

III. **First Aid**
A.   If the cause of the cough is unknown, offer the pet 1/4 cup of prepared chicken bouillon.
B.   If the cough persists, see a veterinarian as soon as possible. Note whether the cough is dry or productive so that your veterinarian can better advise you regarding additional treatment.
C.   If the dog's breathing becomes labored, refer to Breathing Difficulties on page 154.

SYMPTOM – DIARRHEA

I. Problems/Conditions with that Symptom

A. Heat stroke

B. Shock/trauma

C. Infections

D. Poisonings

E. Parasites

F. Cancer

G. Dietary changes or indiscretions

H. Foreign objects

II. First-Aid Materials

A. Kaopectate®

B. Eyedropper or dosage syringe

C. Boiled hamburger and plain cooked rice

III. First Aid

A. If there is no vomiting, feed the dog Kaopectate® using an eyedropper or dosage syringe:

    (1) 1 to 2 teaspoons for dogs weighing less than 20 pounds,

    (2) 3 to 4 teaspoons for dogs weighing 20 or more pounds.

B. Repeat Step A every 4 to 6 hours for adult dogs and every 2 to 4 hours for puppies less than 14 weeks old.

C. Withhold food for 2-4 hours if diarrhea is present and if there is no other symptom of illness. Withhold both food and water if the dog is also vomiting, but do not withhold water for more than 2 hours. Do not withhold water if the dog is not vomiting. The time period for withholding food should be based on whether your pet is a normal, healthy adult versus a puppy, an elderly dog or a dog with any special or compromising conditions. If your dog has diabetes or any other type of illness or medical condition, consult your veterinarian first before withholding food and water.

D. When you do resume feeding your dog, the best home remedy for diarrhea is to prepare a 50/50 mixture of boiled hamburger (drain off the water and fat) and plain cooked rice. Appropriate feedings are as follows:

(1) 1/4 cup of the mixture 4 times per day for small dogs,

(2) 1/2 cup of the mixture 4 times per day for medium dogs,

(3) 3/4 cup of the mixture 4 times per day for large dogs.

Your veterinarian may wish to adjust the servings or may recommend a prescription diet instead.

E. Note the frequency and substance of the diarrhea.

F. If symptoms persist for more than 4 hours, or if they worsen or return, contact the pet's doctor immediately.

SYMPTOM –
DISEMBOWELMENT

I. **Problems/Conditions with that Symptom**

A. Severe trauma

B. Post-operative complications

II. **First-Aid Materials**

A. Towel and/or gauze sponges

B. Contact-lens saline solution

III. **First Aid**

A. Contact a veterinarian immediately.

B. Soak a towel or gauze sponges with saline solution and apply it to the area of protrusion to keep the organs from becoming dehydrated.

C. Keep the organs covered with the wet towel and/or wet sponges to keep the dog from mutilating itself. Dogs will often chew on the bowels if they are exposed.

D. Use an Elizabethan collar if the dog is attempting to chew or scratch the injury. See page 48.

SYMPTOM – DROOLING

I. Problems/Conditions with that Symptom

A. Nausea

B. Gum irritation

C. Diseased teeth

D. Foreign body in mouth

E. Chemical or plant exposure/poisoning

F. Contagious disease (e.g., rabies)

II. First-Aid Materials

A. Pet shampoo

III. First Aid

A. Determine whether your pet may have been exposed to a poison. If so, try to determine the type of poison. Then use the index of this book to find emergency treatment for ingestion of poison in general or, ideally, for ingestion of the particular substance.

B. If there was a flea chemical recently applied to the dog (i.e., that same day), bathe the dog with pet shampoo that does not contain flea chemicals to remove excess chemicals from the coat. Most drooling should stop within 30 minutes.

C. If poisoning or chemicals do not appear to be the cause, check the dog's mouth for diseased teeth, irritated gums and foreign objects by opening the dog's jaws and lifting the dog's lips. (See illustration on page 42.) Do not attempt to remove any object that is wedged in the dog's mouth unless the airway becomes completely blocked; your efforts could injure the dog's mouth or throat. Instead, seek veterinary assistance immediately.

D. If the cause is unknown and the drooling persists, withhold food and water temporarily and contact a veterinarian immediately.

SYMPTOM –
EYES (RUNNY/SORE)

I.   Problems/Conditions with that Symptom

A.   Corneal scratches

B.   Glaucoma

C.   Contusions

D.   Infections

E.   Corneal ulcers

F.   Foreign debris

G.   Allergies

II.   First-Aid Materials

A.   Contact-lens saline solution

III. First Aid

A.   Gently rinse the eye(s) with the contact-lens saline solution by applying several drops to the affected eye. This may dislodge any foreign debris.

B.   If the symptoms improve but reappear, stay the same or worsen, call the dog's veterinarian.

C.   If the dog is rubbing its eye, use an Elizabethan collar to prevent the behavior. See page 48.

D.   Never apply human medicine to a pet's eye unless instructed by a veterinarian.

SYMPTOM – HEAD TILT

The most common cause of a dog having its head tilted is an inner ear problem. Both the underlying condition and the head tilt often result in disorientation, loss of balance and coordination, and sometimes an inability to self-feed.

I. Problems/Conditions with that Symptom

A. Inner ear infections and swelling

B. Trauma

C. Cancers/tumors

D. Foreign body in ear

II. First-Aid Materials

A. Cotton balls

III. First Aid

A. Look in the ear to see if there is a discharge or something blocking the ear canal. Gently wipe any debris from the ear canal using a cotton ball. If the debris is difficult to remove, seek veterinary assistance to prevent further damage and infection.

B. If the dog is disoriented or appears to have a loss of balance or coordination, block off stairways and restrict the pet's activity. Carry or help the dog out to go to the bathroom four times per day.

C. If the dog shows no sign of nausea, offer food and water by hand feeding; the dog's condition may prevent it from eating and drinking out of a bowl.

D. Seek veterinary care as soon as possible.

SYMPTOM – LAMENESS

I.   Problems/Conditions with that Symptom

A.   Fractures

B.   Sprains, torn ligaments and dislocations

C.   Bite wounds

D.   Bruises

E.   Foot-pad injury (e.g., splinter, puncture, laceration)

F.   Torn toenail

G.   Back or neck injury (including slipped disc)

II.   First-Aid Materials

A.   Gauze sponges and roll gauze

B.   Tape

C.   Tweezers

D.   Antibiotic ointment (e.g., Polysporin®)

III.   First Aid

A.   Restrict the dog's activity and try to keep the dog still to prevent further injury.

B.   Use a muzzle to prevent being bitten when treating your dog. However, use a muzzle only if the dog is not having difficulty breathing and has not been vomiting. If at any time the dog has difficulty breathing, remove the muzzle. Also, do not use a muzzle if your dog has a flat face (e.g., a pug, boxer, English bulldog, etc.).

C.   If lameness is caused by a splinter or similar foreign object, use tweezers to remove the object. Apply antibiotic ointment.

D.   For any minor wound where bleeding control is not a problem, apply antibiotic ointment and keep the wound covered with gauze and secure with tape.

E. If the dog has a wound that is bleeding, apply pressure. (For additional information, see Bleeding From Abrasions and Lacerations on page 146.)

F. Monitor the dog's vital signs (temperature, pulse, and respirations).

G. Observe for other injuries.

H. Call a veterinarian for additional instructions.

SYMPTOM – LOSS OF COORDINATION/ LOSS OF BALANCE

Loss of coordination or balance may result from a variety of causes, but one of the most common is an inner ear problem. The inner ear controls balance, posture and head position. If your dog's symptoms are accompanied by a head tilt, then whatever the underlying cause, it is possible there is a problem with the inner ear.

I. Problems/Conditions with that Symptom

A. Inner ear infections and swelling

B. Trauma

C. Cancers/tumors

D. Foreign object in ear

E. Poisoning or extreme illness

II. First-Aid Materials

A. Cotton balls

III. First Aid

A. Look in the ear to see if there is a discharge or something blocking the ear canal. Gently wipe any debris from the ear canal using a cotton ball. If the debris is difficult to remove, seek veterinary assistance to prevent further damage and infection.

B. If the dog is disoriented or appears to have a loss of balance or coordination, block off stairways and restrict the pet's activity. Carry or help the dog out to go to the bathroom four times per day.

C. If the dog shows no sign of nausea, offer food and water by hand feeding; the dog's condition may prevent it from eating and drinking out of a bowl.

D. Seek veterinary care as soon as possible.

SYMPTOM –
PENIS SHEATH DISCHARGE
(BALANOPOSTHITIS)

Inflammation in the sheath surrounding the dog's penis (balanoposthitis) is common and is usually not cause for alarm, but the condition must be treated properly. It may be caused by foreign debris, a laceration, trauma or even a tumor. Dogs are prone to this type of inflammation and infection because there is a natural pocket or cavity in the sheath. When infection occurs, there is generally a cloudy discharge.

I.   Problems/Conditions with that Symptom

A.   Foreign debris in the sheath

B.   Laceration in the penis area

C.   Trauma to the penis/sheath

D.   Tumor in the penis/sheath

II.   First-Aid Materials

A.   Antibiotic ointment (e.g., Polysporin®)

III.   First Aid

A.   Wipe discharge away from sheath.

B.   Apply antibiotic ointment into sheath opening.

C.   Seek veterinary care.

SYMPTOM – PROTRUDING EYE

I. Problems/Conditions with that Symptom

A. Trauma

B. Glaucoma

II. First-Aid Materials

A. Gauze sponges

B. Contact-lens saline solution

III. First Aid

A. Contact a veterinarian immediately.

B. Soak gauze sponge with saline solution and apply to the eye or apply several drops of saline directly onto the affected eye every 5 minutes. This will keep the eye from becoming dehydrated.

C. Do not apply pressure to the eye to stop bleeding.

D. Use an Elizabethan collar if the dog is attempting to scratch at the injury. See page 48.

SYMPTOM – PROTRUDING RECTUM

I.   Problems/Conditions with that Symptom

A.   Diarrhea

B.   Straining

C.   Colitis

D.   Foreign body

II.   First-Aid Materials

A.   Towel and/or gauze sponges

B.   Contact-lens saline solution

C.   Antibiotic ointment (e.g., Polysporin®)

III. First Aid

A.   Contact a veterinarian immediately.

B.   Soak a towel or gauze sponges with saline solution and place on the rectum or apply several drops of saline directly onto the rectum to prevent the organ from becoming dehydrated.

C.   Apply antibiotic ointment to help soothe the discomfort and prevent infection.

D.   An Elizabethan collar may be utilized if the dog is attempting to scratch or chew at the injury. See page 48.

SYMPTOM –
SCRATCHING SKIN/
IRRITATED SKIN

I. Problems/Conditions with that Symptom
A. Contact with plant resins
B. Frostbite
C. Burns
D. Abrasions
E. Bites and stings (e.g., insects, spiders, snakes)
F. Allergies
G. Fleas, lice and/or mites
H. Drug reactions

II. First-Aid Materials
A. Moisturizing shampoo
B. Bath oil (e.g., Alpha Keri®)
C. Elizabethan collar

III. First Aid
A. Shampooing the pet will likely provide temporary relief from its symptoms. Use a shampoo for dogs (moisturizing shampoo is best). While restraining the dog, lather the pet and let stand for 15-20 minutes. Rinse well with warm tap water. Next, mix 1 tablespoon of bath oil (e.g., Alpha Keri®) with 2 quarts of warm tap water. Then pour the bath-oil mixture over the dog's coat, being careful not to get any in its eyes. Let the coat dry naturally. Consult your veterinarian for the proper type of shampoo and for specific instructions.
B. If the dog is biting itself, it may be necessary to apply an Elizabethan collar to prevent more damage to the skin. See page 48 on how to make and use an Elizabethan collar.
C. Seek veterinary help as soon as possible to give more permanent relief from the irritation.

SYMPTOM –
SHAKING HEAD/
SCRATCHING EARS

I. Problems/Conditions with that Symptom
A. Ear infection
B. Ear mites
C. Trauma (physical injury)
D. Bite wounds
E. Ear hematoma (swelling)
F. Toad poisoning

II. First-Aid Materials
A. Gauze sponges or cotton balls

III. First Aid
A. If there is debris in the ear flap, gently remove it by using a dry cotton ball or gauze sponge, being careful not to pack the debris into the ear canal. Do not use water or hydrogen peroxide because the moisture will promote infection.
B. Consult your veterinarian as soon as possible.

SYMPTOM – STRAINING

I. Problems/Conditions with that Symptom

A. Urinary tract irritation or infection

B. Urinary blockage

C. Constipation

D. Colitis

E. Difficult delivery

II. First-Aid Materials

A. 2-liter soda bottle

III. First Aid

A. Observe the dog for urine output. The dog should be able to excrete at least small amounts of urine. If no urine production is detected, it is a life-threatening emergency because the dog may be blocked and unable to urinate.

B. If you suspect urinary blockage proceed as follows:

(1) Contact a veterinarian immediately.

(2) Avoid lifting the dog around its abdomen to prevent discomfort and possible rupture of the bladder.

(3) Keep the dog warm by placing a 2-liter soda bottle filled with warm water (not hot water) against the dog.

(4) Do not encourage the dog to eat or drink because your veterinarian may determine that a urinary catheter is necessary, and insertion of the catheter may require a general anesthetic.

C. Other signs of a urinary tract problem include frequent attempted urination and crying during urination. Even if urine is being produced, if you suspect that there is a urinary tract

175

problem, consult a veterinarian as soon as possible for diagnosis and treatment before the situation turns into a life-threatening block.

D.   If a urinary tract irritation and blockage can be ruled out, see the sections on constipation (page 79), colitis (page 77) and difficult deliveries (page 272).

SYMPTOM –
VOMITING

I. Problems/Conditions with that Symptom

A. Infections

B. Dietary change (e.g., different dog food, table scraps, bones, garbage)

C. Poisonings

D. Heat stroke

E. Shock

F. Foreign objects

G. Organ failure

II. First-Aid Materials

A. Boiled hamburger and plain cooked rice

III. First Aid

A. If the dog is vomiting, withhold food and water for 2-4 hours. (But if your dog has diabetes or any other type of illness or medical condition, consult your veterinarian first before withholding food and water.) Do not withhold food and water from a puppy or elderly dog for more than 2 hours. If symptoms persist, worsen or return within this 2-4 hour period, contact your veterinarian.

B. Note the frequency and substance of the vomiting. Is the food undigested or is the vomitus watery?

C. Note how long after a meal the vomiting occurred.

D. When you do resume feeding your dog, prepare a 50/50 mixture of boiled hamburger (drain off the water and fat) and plain cooked rice. Appropriate feedings are as follows:

(1) 1/4 cup of the mixture 4 times per day for small dogs,

(2) 1/2 cup of the mixture 4 times per day for medium dogs,

(3) 3/4 cup of the mixture 4 times per day for large dogs.

Your veterinarian may wish to adjust the servings or may recommend a prescription diet instead.

E.   Resume normal feeding within 2 days.

SYMPTOM – WEAKNESS/DEPRESSION

Weakness and depression are vague symptoms associated with many diseases and conditions. Recognizing the symptoms is easy, but pinpointing the cause is difficult. Weakness and depression are often early symptoms of a more serious problem.

I. **Problems/Conditions with that Symptom**
A. Heart disease
B. Lung disease
C. Heat stroke
D. Internal bleeding
E. Shock
F. Trauma (physical injury)
G. Anemia
H. Fractured ribs
I. Poisoning
J. Asthma
K. Dehydration
L. Diabetes
M. Liver or kidney disease

II. **First-Aid Materials**
A. Two 2-liter soda bottles
B. Blanket
C. Thermometer

III. **First Aid**
A. Keep the dog calm. Do not use excessive restraint or cause excessive movement.
B. Monitor the dog's vital signs (temperature, pulse, respirations).
C. Keep the dog warm with a blanket and with the 2-liter soda bottles filled with warm water placed close to the dog's body.
D. Call your veterinarian.

SYMPTOM – WETTING IN THE HOUSE

I. Problems/Conditions with that Symptom

A. Urinary-tract irritation or infection

B. Urinary blockage

II. First-Aid Materials

A. 2-liter soda bottle

III. First Aid

A. Observe the dog for urine output. The dog should be able to excrete at least small amounts of urine. If no urine production is detected, it is a life-threatening emergency because the dog may be blocked and unable to urinate.

B. If you suspect urinary blockage, proceed as follows:

(1) Contact a veterinarian immediately.

(2) Avoid lifting the dog around its abdomen to prevent discomfort and possible rupture of the bladder.

(3) Keep the dog warm by placing a 2-liter soda bottle filled with warm water (not hot water) against the dog.

(4) Do not encourage the dog to eat or drink because your veterinarian may determine that a urinary catheter is necessary, and insertion of the catheter may require a general anesthetic.

C. Other signs of a urinary tract problem include straining, frequent attempted urination and crying during urination. Even if urine is being produced, if you suspect that there is a urinary tract problem, consult a veterinarian as soon as possible for diagnosis and treatment before the situation turns into a life-threatening block.

PART 4

—

POISON BASICS

GENERAL PROCEDURES

Because some poisons are sweet to the taste and because of the inherent curiosity of most dogs, poisons pose a substantial risk to your pet. Early recognition is critical to prevent complications or death.

I. Information About the Dog

A. Be ready to provide the following information to your veterinarian: owner's name, address and phone number and the dog's breed, age, sex and weight.

B. If you have more than one pet, note whether the others are affected.

C. Be able to describe the symptoms the dog is experiencing.

II. Information About the Exposure

A. Note the suspected substance.

B. Identify the substance ingested. Save the label or container of the suspected agent, if applicable. If the agent is a plant and cannot be identified, obtain a sample of the plant.

C. Note the time of exposure.

D. Note the amount of the substance ingested.

III. Steps to Get Help

A. Immediately contact the dog's veterinarian to see if treatment is necessary.

B. If you cannot reach a veterinarian, call the National Animal Poison Control Center for information (for a fee of $20 for five minutes at the time of this printing: 1-900-680-0000) or a local poison control hotline.

C. Follow the veterinarian's or the Center's recommendations.

D. If you need to induce vomiting, see page 40.

E. Observe for symptoms (vomiting, diarrhea, loss of coordination, lethargy, etc.). Symptoms may not be evident immediately.

LIST OF COMMON POISONS

I. List of Common Poisons (see note at bottom of list)

Acetaminophen*
Adhesives
Amphetamines
Antidepressants
Antihistamines
Arsenic*
Barbiturates
Bleach
Bromethalin
Carbon monoxide
Chocolate*
Coal tar
Creosote
DEET
Drain cleaners
Ethylene glycol*
Flea products*
Glue
Insulin
Ivermectin
Limonene
Metaldehyde
Methylxanthines
Narcotic analgesics
Petroleum distillates*
Phenylpropanolamine
Propranolol
Rat poison*
Strychnine*

Acids*
Alkalis*
Antidandruff shampoos
Antifreeze*
Antipsychotics
Atropine
Benzodiazepines
Borates
Camphor
Chlorinated hydrocarbons
Cholecalciferol
Cocaine
Cyanide
Detergents
Ethanol
5-fluorouracil
4-animopyridine
Ibuprofen*
Isopropanol
Lead*
Mercury
Methanol
Naphthaline
PCP
Phenols
Pine oil
Pyrethrins
Snail bait*
1080

Terbutaline   THC

2,4-D   Xanthines

Zinc oxide

*See Part 6 starting on page 238 for more details.

NOTE: The above list does not include all poisons. Some substances that are not harmful to people are poisonous to dogs. Many common household products contain chemicals that are poisonous to dogs. It is reasonable to assume that anything that is poisonous to people is likely poisonous to dogs. For plant poisons, see Part 5 of this book starting on page 186.

PART 5

—

POISONOUS PLANTS

INTRODUCTION TO POISONOUS PLANTS

Many plant poisonings require quick home treatment followed by immediate veterinary care. Veterinary follow-up is critical to prevent secondary effects of the poisons. Also, a veterinarian can monitor the dog for complications.

It is important to note that because of the huge number of plants in existence, this section of this book cannot possibly address every plant that is or may be toxic to dogs. Also, some plants that are generally considered to be nontoxic may cause severe symptoms in a dog with an allergy to the plant. And some plants that are not toxic are sprayed with chemicals that may be poisonous. Therefore, you should be concerned whenever your dog eats any type of plant, and you should contact your veterinarian immediately.

ALOCASIA

I. **Toxic Portion of Plant**
- A.   All parts

II. **Symptoms (one or both may be present)**
- A.   Digestive upset
- B.   Burning sensation in mouth

III. **First Aid**
- A.   Feed milk to your dog.
- B.   Call your veterinarian immediately.
- C.   Observe for symptoms.

ALOE VERA

I. **Toxic Portion of Plant**
- A.   All parts

II. **Symptoms (one or both may be present)**
- A.   Diarrhea
- B.   Urine may turn red in color

III. **First Aid**
- A.   If your dog is alert, induce vomiting.
- B.   Call your veterinarian immediately.
- C.   Observe for symptoms.

AMARYLLIS (Hippeastrum)

I. **Toxic Portion of Plant**
- A.   Bulb is most toxic.

II. **Symptoms (some or all may be present)**
- A.   Digestive upset
- B.   Excitement followed by depression, then coma
- C.   Possible death

III. **First Aid**
- A.   If your dog is alert, induce vomiting.

B.   Call your veterinarian immediately.

C.   Observe for symptoms.

APPLE (Malus)

I.   Toxic Portion of Plant

A.   Leaves and stems contain cyanide.

B.   Dried, withering leaves are most toxic.

II.   Symptoms (some or all may be present)

A.   Rapid breathing

B.   Dilated pupils

C.   Red gums

D.   Shock

III.   First Aid

A.   If your dog is alert, induce vomiting.

B.   Call your veterinarian immediately.

C.   Observe for symptoms.

AUTUMN CROCUS (Colchicum)

I.   Toxic Portion of Plant

A.   Mostly bulbs

II.   Symptoms (some or all may be present)

A.   Oral irritation

B.   Digestive upset

C.   Kidney failure

D.   Excitement followed by depression, then coma – may begin approximately 8 hours after ingestion

E.   Shock with possible death – following initial onset of other symptoms

III.   First Aid

A.   If your dog is alert, induce vomiting.

B.   Call your veterinarian immediately.

C.   Observe for symptoms.

AVOCADO (Persea americana)

I. **Toxic Portion of Plant**
   A. Seed
II. **Symptoms (some or all may be present)**
   A. Vomiting
   B. Diarrhea
   C. Difficulty breathing
   D. Possible death
III. **First Aid**
   A. If your dog is alert, induce vomiting.
   B. Call your veterinarian immediately.
   C. Observe for symptoms.

AZALEA (Rhododendron)

I. **Toxic Portion of Plant**
   A. All parts
II. **Symptoms (some or all may be present)**
   A. Digestive upset
   B. Heart failure
   C. Depression
   D. Drooling
   E. Weakness
   F. Coma
III. **First Aid**
   A. If your dog is alert, induce vomiting.
   B. Call your veterinarian immediately.
   C. Observe for symptoms.

BIRD-OF-PARADISE (Strelitzia reginae)

I. **Toxic Portion of Plant**
   A. Seed pod
II. **Symptoms (one or both may be present)**

A. Digestive upset

B. Disoriented walking (occurs within 30 minutes)

III. First Aid

A. Induce vomiting if ingestion was within 1 hour and your dog is alert.

B. If ingestion of plant occurred more that 60 minutes prior, feed milk to the dog.

C. Call your veterinarian immediately.

D. Observe for symptoms.

BLACK LOCUST (Rubinia pseudoacacia)

I. Toxic Portion of Plant

A. Bark

B. Green growth

C. Seeds

II. Symptoms (some or all may be present)

A. Digestive upset

B. Heart failure

C. Depression

III. First Aid

A. If your dog is alert, induce vomiting.

B. Call your veterinarian immediately.

C. Observe for symptoms.

BLEEDING-HEART (Dicentra)

I. Toxic Portion of Plant

A. Top growth

B. Corms

II. Symptoms (some or all may be present)

A. Digestive upset

B. Irritation of mouth with possible swelling of the throat

C. Possible asphyxiation

D. Central nervous system signs - tremors, seizures,

190

staggering, loss of coordination, etc.

    E.   Possible death

III. First Aid

    A.   If your dog is alert, induce vomiting.

    B.   Call your veterinarian immediately.

    C.   Observe for symptoms.

BOXWOOD (Buxus)

I.   Toxic Portion of Plant

    A.   All parts

II. Symptoms (some or all may be present)

    A.   Digestive upset

    B.   Excitement or depression

    C.   Heart failure

III. First Aid

    A.   If your dog is alert, induce vomiting.

    B.   Call your veterinarian immediately.

    C.   Observe for symptoms.

BROAD BEAN (Vicia faba)

See Fava Bean on page 205.

BUCKEYE (Aesculus)

I.   Toxic Portion of Plant

    A.   Seed

II. Symptoms (some or all may be present)

    A.   Digestive upset

    B.   Depression or excitement

    C.   Dilated pupils

    D.   Paralysis

    E.   Coma with possible death

III. First Aid
   A. If your dog is alert, induce vomiting.
   B. Call your veterinarian immediately.
   C. Observe for symptoms.

BUDDHIST PINE (Podocarpus)

I. Toxic Portion of Plant
   A. All parts
II. Symptom
   A. Severe digestive upset
III. First Aid
   A. If your dog is alert, induce vomiting.
   B. Call your veterinarian immediately.
   C. Observe for symptoms.

BUTTERCUP (Ranunculus)

I. Toxic Portion of Plant
   A. Top growth
II. Symptom
   A. Digestive upset
III. First Aid
   A. If your dog is alert, induce vomiting.
   B. Call your veterinarian immediately.
   C. Observe for symptoms.

CALADIUM

I. Toxic Portion of Plant
   A. Leaves
   B. Stems
   C. Stalks
   D. Plant cells contain toxic calcium oxalate crystals.

II. Symptoms (some or all may be present)

A. Digestive upset

B. Irritation of mouth with possible swelling of the throat

C. Possible asphyxiation

D. Central nervous system signs - tremors, seizures, staggering, loss of coordination, etc.

E. Possible death

III. First Aid

A. If your dog is alert, induce vomiting.

B. Call your veterinarian immediately.

C. Observe for symptoms.

CALAMONDIN ORANGE (Citrus mitis)

I. Toxic Portion of Plant

A. Leaves

B. Stems

C. Stalks

D. Plant cells contain toxic calcium oxalate crystals.

II. Symptoms (some or all may be present)

A. Digestive upset

B. Irritation of mouth with possible swelling of the throat

C. Possible asphyxiation

D. Central nervous system signs - tremors, seizures, staggering, loss of coordination, etc.

E. Possible death

III. First Aid

A. If your dog is alert, induce vomiting.

B. Call your veterinarian immediately.

C. Observe for symptoms.

CALLA LILY (Zantedeschia)

I. Toxic Portion of Plant

A. Leaves

193

B. Stems

C. Stalks

D. Plant cells contain toxic calcium oxalate crystals.

II. Symptoms (some or all may be present)

A. Digestive upset

B. Irritation of mouth with possible swelling of the throat

C. Possible asphyxiation

D. Central nervous system signs - tremors, seizures, staggering, loss of coordination, etc.

E. Possible death

III. First Aid

A. If your dog is alert, induce vomiting.

B. Call your veterinarian immediately.

C. Observe for symptoms.

CASTOR BEAN (Ricinus communis)

I. Toxic Portion of Plant

A. All parts

B. Seeds are especially toxic.

C. One leaf or seed may be deadly.

II. Symptoms (some or all may be present)

A. Digestive upset

B. Excess thirst

C. Irritation of mouth and throat

D. Liver and kidney damage

E. Central nervous system signs - tremors, staggering, loss of coordination, etc.

F. Seizures

G. Possible death

III. First Aid

A. If your dog is alert, induce vomiting.

B. Call your veterinarian immediately.

C. Observe for symptoms.

CERIMAN (Monstera deliciosa)

See Philodendron on page 224.

CHARMING DIEFFENBACHIA (Dieffenbachia amoena)

See Dumb Cane on page 202.

CHERRY (Prunus)

I. **Toxic Portion of Plant**

    A. Leaves and stems contain cyanide.

    B. Dried, withering leaves are most toxic.

II. **Symptoms (some or all may be present)**

    A. Rapid breathing

    B. Dilated pupils

    C. Red gums

    D. Shock

III. **First Aid**

    A. If your dog is alert, induce vomiting.

    B. Call your veterinarian immediately.

    C. Observe for symptoms.

CHRISTMAS ROSE (Helleborus niger)

I. **Toxic Portion of Plant**

    A. All parts

II. **Symptoms (some or all may be present)**

    A. Digestive upset

    B. Bloody diarrhea

    C. Seizures

    D. Disorientation

III. **First Aid**

    A. If your dog is alert, induce vomiting.

B. Call your veterinarian immediately.

C. Observe for symptoms.

CHRYSANTHEMUM

I. Toxic Portion of Plant

A. All parts

II. Symptom

A. Irritation of mucus membranes and any skin that comes in contact with the plant's resin.

III. First Aid

A. Feed milk to your dog.

B. Wash irritated skin with soap and water.

C. Call your veterinarian immediately.

D. Observe for symptoms.

CINERARIA (Senecio)

I. Toxic Portion of Plant

A. All parts

II. Symptoms (some or all may be present)

A. Digestive upset

B. Depression

C. Dark/muddy gum color

D. Liver damage

III. First Aid

A. If your dog is alert, induce vomiting.

B. Call your veterinarian immediately.

C. Observe for symptoms.

COLOCASIA

See Elephant's Ear on page 204.

CORDATUM (Philodendron oxycardium)

I. **Toxic Portion of Plant**

    A.   Leaves

    B.   Stems

    C.   Stalks

    D.   Plant cells contain toxic calcium oxalate crystals.

II. **Symptoms (some or all may be present)**

    A.   Digestive upset

    B.   Irritation of mouth with possible swelling of the throat

    C.   Possible asphyxiation

    D.   Central nervous system signs - tremors, seizures, staggering, loss of coordination, etc.

    E.   Possible death

III. **First Aid**

    A.   If your dog is alert, induce vomiting.

    B.   Call your veterinarian immediately.

    C.   Observe for symptoms.

CORN (CORNSTALK) PLANT (Dracaena fragrans massangeana)

I. **Toxic Portion of Plant**

    A.   All parts

II. **Symptoms (some or all may be present)**

    A.   Digestive upset

    B.   Dilated pupils

    C.   Difficult breathing

    D.   Drooling

    E.   Abdominal pain

III. **First Aid**

    A.   If your dog is alert, induce vomiting.

    B.   Call your veterinarian immediately.

    C.   Observe for symptoms.

CORYDALIS

I. Toxic Portion of Plant
    A. Top growth
    B. Corms

II. Symptoms (some or all may be present)
    A. Digestive upset
    B. Irritation of mouth with possible swelling of the throat
    C. Possible asphyxiation
    D. Central nervous system signs - tremors, seizures, staggering, loss of coordination, etc.
    E. Possible death

III. First Aid
    A. If your dog is alert, induce vomiting.
    B. Call your veterinarian immediately.
    C. Observe for symptoms.

CROTALARIA

I. Toxic Portion of Plant
    A. Seeds (plus other parts may also cause a toxic reaction)

II. Symptoms (some or all may be present)
    A. Liver damage
    B. Digestive upset
    C. Birth defects in offspring

III. First Aid
    A. If your dog is alert, induce vomiting.
    B. Call your veterinarian immediately.
    C. Observe for symptoms.

CROTON

I. Toxic Portion of Plant
    A. All parts
    B. Seeds are especially toxic.

C.   One leaf or seed may be deadly.

II.   Symptoms (some or all may be present)

A.   Digestive upset

B.   Liver and kidney damage

C.   Central nervous system signs - tremors, seizures, staggering, loss of coordination, etc.

D.   Possible death

III.   First Aid

A.   If your dog is alert, induce vomiting.

B.   Call your veterinarian immediately.

C.   Observe for symptoms.

CROWFOOT FAMILY

See Buttercup on page 192.

CROWN OF THORNS (Euphorbia milii)

I.   Toxic Portion of Plant

A.   All parts

II.   Symptoms (one or both may be present)

A.   Digestive upset

B.   Skin irritation

III.   First Aid

A.   If your dog is alert, induce vomiting.

B.   Call your veterinarian immediately.

C.   Observe for symptoms.

CUBAN LAUREL (Ficus)

I.   Toxic Portion of Plant

A.   All parts

II.   Symptom

A.   Digestive upset

III. First Aid

    A. If your dog is alert, induce vomiting.

    B. Call your veterinarian immediately.

    C. Observe for symptoms.

CYCAD (Cycas)

I. Toxic Portion of Plant

    A. All parts

II. Symptoms (some or all may be present)

    A. Digestive upset

    B. Black stools

    C. Internal bleeding

    D. Bruising

    E. Liver damage and jaundice - yellow hue to skin and gums

III. First Aid

    A. If your dog is alert, induce vomiting.

    B. Call your veterinarian immediately.

    C. Observe for symptoms.

CYCLAMEN

I. Toxic Portion of Plant

    A. All parts

II. Symptoms (one or both may be present)

    A. Digestive upset

    B. Death

III. First Aid

    A. If your dog is alert, induce vomiting.

    B. Call your veterinarian immediately.

    C. Observe for symptoms.

DAFFODIL (Narcissus)

I. **Toxic Portion of Plant**
   A.   Bulb is most toxic.
II. **Symptoms (some or all may be present)**
   A.   Digestive upset
   B.   Seizures
   C.   Shaking
   D.   Weakness
   E.   Irregular heart beats
   F.   Excitement followed by depression, then coma
   G.   Possible death
III. **First Aid**
   A.   If your dog is alert, induce vomiting.
   B.   Call your veterinarian immediately.
   C.   Observe for symptoms.

DAPHNE

I. **Toxic Portion of Plant**
   A.   All parts
II. **Symptoms (some or all may be present)**
   A.   Digestive upset
   B.   Heart failure
   C.   Excitement or depression
III. **First Aid**
   A.   If your dog is alert, induce vomiting.
   B.   Call your veterinarian immediately.
   C.   Observe for symptoms.

DEATH CAMAS (Zigadenus)

I. **Toxic Portion of Plant**
   A.   Bulb is most toxic.
II. **Symptoms (some or all may be present)**

A. Digestive upset

B. Excitement followed by depression, then coma

C. Possible death

III. **First Aid**

A. If your dog is alert, induce vomiting.

B. Call your veterinarian immediately.

C. Observe for symptoms.

DEVIL'S IVY

See Philodendron on page 224.

DRACAENA PALM

See Corn Plant on page 197.

DRAGON TREE (Dracaena draco)

See Corn Plant on page 197.

DUMB CANE (DIEFFENBACHIA)

I. **Toxic Portion of Plant**

A. Leaves

B. Stems

C. Stalks

D. Plant cells contain toxic calcium oxalate crystals.

II. **Symptoms (some or all may be present)**

A. Digestive upset

B. Irritation of mouth with possible swelling of the throat

C. Possible asphyxiation

D. Central nervous system signs - tremors, seizures, staggering, loss of coordination, etc.

E. Possible death

III. **First Aid**

A. If your dog is alert, induce vomiting.

B.   Call your veterinarian immediately.

C.   Observe for symptoms.

EASTER LILY (Lilium longiflorum)

I.   Toxic Portion of Plant

A.   All parts

II.   Symptoms (some or all may be present)

A.   Kidney failure

B.   Digestive upset

C.   Weakness

III.   First Aid

A.   If your dog is alert, induce vomiting.

B.   Call your veterinarian immediately.

C.   Observe for symptoms.

EGGPLANT

I.   Toxic Portion of Plant

A.   Leaves

B.   Stems

C.   Stalks

D.   Sprouts

E.   Fruit is edible.

II.   Symptoms (some or all may be present)

A.   Digestive upset

B.   Heart failure

C.   Depression/drowsiness

D.   Drooling

E.   Dilated pupils

III.   First Aid

A.   If your dog is alert, induce vomiting.

B.   Call your veterinarian immediately.

C.   Observe for symptoms.

ELAINE CODIAEUM (Elaine)

See Croton on page 198.

ELEPHANT'S EAR (Colocasia esculenta)

I. **Toxic Portion of Plant**
    A. Leaves
    B. Stems
    C. Stalks
    D. Plant cells contain toxic calcium oxalate crystals.
II. **Symptoms (some or all may be present)**
    A. Digestive upset
    B. Irritation of mouth with possible swelling of the throat
    C. Possible asphyxiation
    D. Central nervous system signs - tremors, seizures, staggering, loss of coordination, etc.
    E. Possible death
III. **First Aid**
    A. If your dog is alert, induce vomiting.
    B. Call your veterinarian immediately.
    C. Observe for symptoms.

EMERALD FEATHER (Asparagus sprengeri)

See Asparagus Fern on page 235.

ENGLISH IVY (Hedera helix)

I. **Toxic Portion of Plant**
    A. All parts
    B. Contains a saponic glycoside
II. **Symptoms (some or all may be present)**
    A. Digestive upset

B.   Excitability

C.   Difficult breathing

D.   Drooling

E.   Fever

F.   Increased thirst

G.   Dilated pupils

H.   Weakness

I.   Staggering

III. **First Aid**

A.   If your dog is alert, induce vomiting.

B.   Call your veterinarian immediately.

C.   Observe for symptoms.

EXOTICA PERFECTION DIEFFENBACHIA (Dieffenbachia exotica)

See Dumb Cane on page 202.

FAVA BEAN (Vicia faba)

I.   **Toxic Portion of Plant**

A.   Seeds (plus other parts may also cause a toxic reaction)

II. **Symptoms (some or all may be present)**

A.   Liver damage

B.   Digestive upset

C.   Birth defects in offspring

III. **First Aid**

A.   If your dog is alert, induce vomiting.

B.   Call your veterinarian immediately.

C.   Observe for symptoms.

FIDDLE-LEAF FIG (Ficus lyrata)

I.   **Toxic Portion of Plant**

A. All parts
II. **Symptoms (one or both may be present)**
   A. Skin irritation in some dogs upon contact
   B. Digestive upset
III. **First Aid**
   A. If your dog is alert, induce vomiting.
   B. Call your veterinarian immediately.
   C. Observe for symptoms.

FINGER CHERRY (Rhodomyrtus macrocarpa)

I. **Toxic Portion of Plant**
   A. Fruit
II. **Symptom**
   A. Blindness (may be complete and permanent)
III. **First Aid**
   A. If your dog is alert, induce vomiting.
   B. Call your veterinarian immediately.
   C. Observe for symptoms.

FLORIDA BEAUTY (Dracaena)

See Corn Plant on page 197.

FOXGLOVE (Digitalis)

I. **Toxic Portion of Plant**
   A. All parts
   B. Seeds especially
II. **Symptoms (some or all may be present)**
   A. Digestive upset
   B. Central nervous system signs - tremors, seizures, staggering, loss of coordination, etc.

206

C. Depression
D. Collapse
E. Heart failure
F. Possible death

III. First Aid
A. If your dog is alert, induce vomiting.
B. Call your veterinarian immediately.
C. Observe for symptoms.

FRUIT-SALAD PLANT (Monstera deliciosa)

See Philodendron on page 224.

GERMAN IVY (Senecio mikanioides)

See Cineraria on page 196.

GIANT DUMB CANE (Dieffenbachia amoena)

See Dumb Cane on page 202.

GLACIER IVY (Hedera helix glacier)

See English Ivy on page 204.

GOLD DIEFFENBACHIA (Dieffenbachia picta rudolph roehrs)

See Dumb Cane on page 202.

GOLD DUST DRACAENA (Dracaena godseffiana)

See Corn Plant on page 197.

GOLDEN POTHOS (Epipremnum aureum)

See Philodendron on page 224.

GREEN GOLD NEPHTHYTIS (Syngonium podophyllum)

See Philodendron on page 224.

GROUND CHERRY

I. **Toxic Portion of Plant**
    A. Leaves
    B. Stems
    C. Stalks
    D. Sprouts
    E. Fruit is edible.

II. **Symptoms (some or all may be present)**
    A. Digestive upset
    B. Drowsiness
    C. Weakness
    D. Drooling
    E. Shaking
    F. Paralysis
    G. Coma

III. **First Aid**
    A. If your dog is alert, induce vomiting.
    B. Call your veterinarian immediately.
    C. Observe for symptoms.

HEMLOCK (Conium maculatum)

I.   **Toxic Portion of Plant**
     A.   All parts
II. **Symptoms (some or all may be present)**
     A.   Central nervous system signs - tremors, seizures, staggering, loss of coordination, etc.
     B.   Depression
III. **First Aid**
     A.   If your dog is alert, induce vomiting.
     B.   Call your veterinarian immediately.
     C.   Observe for symptoms.

HOLLY (Ilex)

I.   **Toxic Portion of Plant**
     A.   Berries
II. **Symptoms (one or both may be present)**
     A.   Digestive upset
     B.   Central nervous system depression
III. **First Aid**
     A.   If your dog is alert, induce vomiting.
     B.   Call your veterinarian immediately.
     C.   Observe for symptoms.

HORSE BEAN (Vicia faba)

See Fava Bean on page 205.

HORSEHEAD PHILODENDRON (Philodendron bipinnatifidum)

See Philodendron on page 224.

HURRICANE PLANT (Monstera deliciosa)

See Philodendron on page 224.

HYDRANGEA

I. **Toxic Portion of Plant**
  A. All parts
  B. Plants contain cyanide properties.

II. **Symptoms (some or all may be present)**
  A. Dizziness
  B. Increased breathing
  C. Seizures

III. **First Aid**
  A. If your dog is alert, induce vomiting.
  B. Call your veterinarian immediately.
  C. Observe for symptoms.

INDIAN LAUREL (Ficus retusa nitida)

See Fiddle-leaf Fig on page 205.

INDIAN TOBACCO (Lobelia inflata)

I. **Toxic Portion of Plant**
  A. All parts

II. **Symptoms (some or all may be present)**
  A. Digestive upset
  B. Tremors
  C. Stupor
  D. Constricted pupils
  E. Depression

III. **First Aid**
  A. If your dog is alert, induce vomiting.
  B. Call your veterinarian immediately.

C.   Observe for symptoms.

INDIA RUBBER PLANT (Ficus elastica decora)
See Fiddle-leaf Fig on page 205.

IRIS
I.   **Toxic Portion of Plant**
    A.   Root
II. **Symptom**
    A.   Digestive upset
III. **First Aid**
    A.   If your dog is alert, induce vomiting.
    B.   Call your veterinarian immediately.
    C.   Observe for symptoms.

JANET CRAIG DRACAENA (Dracaena deremensis Janet Craig)
See Corn Plant on page 197.

JAPANESE YEW (Taxus cuspidata)
I.   **Toxic Portion of Plant**
    A.   All parts
    B.   Berries
II. **Symptoms (some or all may be present)**
    A.   Digestive upset
    B.   Heart failure
    C.   Shaking
    D.   Difficult breathing
    E.   Excitement or depression

III. First Aid

    A.   If your dog is alert, induce vomiting.

    B.   Call your veterinarian immediately.

    C.   Observe for symptoms.

JAVA BEAN

I. Toxic Portion of Plant

    A.   Seeds (plus other parts may also cause a toxic reaction)

II. Symptoms (some or all may be present)

    A.   Liver damage

    B.   Digestive upset

    C.   Birth defects in offspring

III. First Aid

    A.   If your dog is alert, induce vomiting.

    B.   Call your veterinarian immediately.

    C.   Observe for symptoms.

JERUSALEM CHERRY (Solanum pseudocapsicum)

I. Toxic Portion of Plant

    A.   Berries (plus other parts may also cause a toxic reaction)

II. Symptoms (some or all may be present)

    A.   Digestive upset

    B.   Ulceration of the digestive tract

    C.   Seizures

    D.   Depression

    E.   Shaking

    F.   Drooling

    G.   Paralysis

    H.   Coma

III. First Aid

    A.   If your dog is alert, induce vomiting.

B.   Call your veterinarian immediately.

C.   Observe for symptoms.

JESSAMINE (Jasminum)

I.   **Toxic Portion of Plant**

    A.   All parts

II.   **Symptoms (some or all may be present)**

    A.   Weakness

    B.   Seizures

    C.   Difficult breathing and/or respiratory failure

III. **First Aid**

    A.   If your dog is alert, induce vomiting.

    B.   Call your veterinarian immediately.

    C.   Observe for symptoms.

JIMSONWEED (Datura stramonium)

I.   **Toxic Portion of Plant**

    A.   All parts

    B.   Seeds are especially toxic.

II.   **Symptoms (some or all may be present)**

    A.   Digestive upset

    B.   Disorientation

    C.   Abnormal thirst

    D.   Coma

    E.   Possible death

III. **First Aid**

    A.   If your dog is alert, induce vomiting.

    B.   Call your veterinarian immediately.

    C.   Observe for symptoms.

JONQUIL (Narcissus jonquilla)

I. **Toxic Portion of Plant**

    A.   Bulb is most toxic.

II. **Symptoms (some or all may be present)**

    A.   Digestive upset

    B.   Excitement followed by depression, then coma

    C.   Possible death

III. **First Aid**

    A.   If your dog is alert, induce vomiting.

    B.   Call your veterinarian immediately.

    C.   Observe for symptoms.

KALANCHOE

I. **Toxic Portion of Plant**

    A.   All parts

II. **Symptom**

    A.   Digestive upset

III. **First Aid**

    A.   If your dog is alert, induce vomiting.

    B.   Call your veterinarian immediately.

    C.   Observe for symptoms.

LACY TREE PHILODENDRON (Philodendron selloum)

See Philodendron on page 224.

LARKSPUR (Delphinium)

I. **Toxic Portion of Plant**

    A.   Flowers

    B.   Seeds

II. **Symptoms (some or all may be present)**
   A. Digestive upset
   B. Central nervous system signs - tremors, seizures, staggering, loss of coordination, etc.
   C. Depression
   D. Collapse
   E. Heart failure
   F. Possible death
III. **First Aid**
   A. If your dog is alert, induce vomiting.
   B. Call your veterinarian immediately.
   C. Observe for symptoms.

LAUREL

I. **Toxic Portion of Plant**
   A. All parts
II. **Symptoms (some or all may be present)**
   A. Digestive upset
   B. Tearing
   C. Discharge from nose
   D. Drooling
   E. Seizures
   F. Slow heart rate
   G. Paralysis
III. **First Aid**
   A. If your dog is alert, induce vomiting.
   B. Call your veterinarian immediately.
   C. Observe for symptoms.

LILY OF THE VALLEY (Convallaria majalis)

I. **Toxic Portion of Plant**

A. Bulb is most toxic.

II. Symptoms (some or all may be present)
A. Digestive upset
B. Excitement followed by depression, then coma
C. Staggering
D. Irregular heartbeat
E. Possible death

III. First Aid
A. If your dog is alert, induce vomiting.
B. Call your veterinarian immediately.
C. Observe for symptoms.

LOCO WEEDS

I. Toxic Portion of Plant
A. Seeds (plus other parts may also cause a toxic reaction)

II. Symptoms (some or all may be present)
A. Liver damage
B. Digestive upset
C. Central nervous system signs - tremors, seizures, staggering, loss of coordination, etc.
D. Birth defects in offspring

III. First Aid
A. If your dog is alert, induce vomiting.
B. Call your veterinarian immediately.
C. Observe for symptoms.

LUPINES

I. Toxic Portion of Plant
A. Berries (plus other parts may also cause a toxic reaction)

II. Symptoms (some or all may be present)
A. Liver damage
B. Digestive upset
C. Birth defects in offspring

216

D. Paralysis

E. Seizures

F. Depressed breathing

III. First Aid

A. If your dog is alert, induce vomiting.

B. Call your veterinarian immediately.

C. Observe for symptoms.

MADAGASCAR DRAGON TREE (Dracaena marginata)

See Corn Plant on page 197.

MANCHINEEL (Hippomane mancinella)

I. Toxic Portion of Plant

A. Sap (found in all plant parts)

B. Fruit

II. Symptoms (one or both may be present)

A. Skin irritation from contact with the sap

B. Severe digestive problems (from fruit especially)

III. First Aid

A. Feed milk to your dog if your dog has ingested the plant.

B. Wash any irritated skin with soap and water.

C. Call your veterinarian immediately.

D. Observe for symptoms.

MARBLE QUEEN (Scindapsus aureus Marble Queen)

I. Toxic Portion of Plant
A. All parts

II. Symptoms (some or all may be present)

A. Digestive upset

B. Depression

C. Respiratory depression

III. **First Aid**

    A. If your dog is alert, induce vomiting.

    B. Call your veterinarian immediately.

    C. Observe for symptoms.

MARIJUANA (Cannabis sativa)

I. **Toxic Portion of Plant**

    A. All parts

II. **Symptoms (some or all may be present)**

    A. Digestive upset

    B. Depression

    C. Respiratory depression

III. **First Aid**

    A. If your dog is alert, induce vomiting.

    B. Call your veterinarian immediately.

    C. Observe for symptoms.

MAY APPLE (Podophyllum peltatum)

I. **Toxic Portion of Plant**

    A. Roots

II. **Symptoms (some or all may be present)**

    A. Digestive upset

    B. Depression

    C. Exhaustion

    D. Coma

    E. Possible death

III. **First Aid**

    A. If your dog is alert, induce vomiting.

    B. Call your veterinarian immediately.

    C. Observe for symptoms.

MEDICINE PLANT (Aloe vera)

I. **Toxic Portion of Plant**

    A.   All parts

II. **Symptoms (one or both may be present)**

    A.   Diarrhea

    B.   Urine may turn red

III. **First Aid**

    A.   If your dog is alert, induce vomiting.

    B.   Call your veterinarian immediately.

    C.   Observe for symptoms.

MISTLETOE (Phoradendron flavescens)

I. **Toxic Portion of Plant**

    A.   All parts

    B.   Seeds are especially toxic.

II. **Symptoms (some or all may be present)**

    A.   Digestive upset

    B.   Depression

    C.   Heart failure

    D.   Exhaustion

    E.   Coma

    F.   Possible death

III. **First Aid**

    A.   If your dog is alert, induce vomiting.

    B.   Call your veterinarian immediately.

    C.   Observe for symptoms.

MONKSHOOD (Aconitum)

I. **Toxic Portion of Plant**

    A.   Flowers

    B.   Seeds

II. **Symptoms (some or all may be present)**

A. Digestive upset

B. Central nervous system signs - tremors, seizures, staggering, loss of coordination, etc.

C. Depression

D. Collapse

E. Heart failure

F. Possible death

III. First Aid

A. If your dog is alert, induce vomiting.

B. Call your veterinarian immediately.

C. Observe for symptoms.

MORNING GLORY (Ipomoea)

I. Toxic Portion of Plant

A. All parts

B. Seeds contain LSD-like compounds.

II. Symptoms (one or both may be present)

A. Digestive upset

B. Hallucinations

III. First Aid

A. If your dog is alert, induce vomiting.

B. Call your veterinarian immediately.

C. Observe for symptoms.

MOTHER-IN-LAW PLANT (Dieffenbachia)

See Dumb Cane on page 202.

MUSHROOMS

I. Toxicity

A. Many species of mushrooms and toadstools are poisonous, especially the Amanita species.

II. Symptoms (some or all may be present)

    A.   Digestive upset

    B.   Drooling

    C.   Constricted or dilated pupils

    D.   Shaking/shivering/muscle spasms

    E.   Weakness

    F.   Irregular heartbeat

    G.   Liver damage

    H.   Possible blood in urine

    I.   Possible coma and death

III. First Aid

    A.   Identify the mushroom the dog has ingested. If the mushroom cannot be identified, obtain a sample of the fungus. Plants can be identified by veterinarians and by plant identification books.

    B.   If you suspect that the mushroom is poisonous and your dog is alert, induce vomiting and call a veterinarian.

    C.   Observe for symptoms.

NARCISSUS

I. Toxic Portion of Plant

    A.   Bulb is most toxic.

II. Symptoms (some or all may be present)

    A.   Digestive upset

    B.   Excitement followed by depression, then coma

    C.   Seizures

    D.   Shaking/shivering

    E.   Weakness

    F.   Irregular heartbeat

    G.   Possible death

III. First Aid

    A.   If your dog is alert, induce vomiting.

    B.   Call your veterinarian immediately.

    C.   Observe for symptoms.

NEEDLEPOINT IVY (Hedera helix needlepoint)

See English Ivy on page 204.

NIGHTSHADE (Solanum)

I. **Toxic Portion of Plant**
   A. All parts
   B. Berries are also toxic.
II. **Symptoms (some or all may be present)**
   A. Digestive upset
   B. Heart failure
   C. Depression/drowsiness
   D. Drooling
   E. Dilated pupils
III. **First Aid**
   A. If your dog is alert, induce vomiting.
   B. Call your veterinarian immediately.
   C. Observe for symptoms.

OLEANDER (Nerium oleander)

I. **Toxic Portion of Plant**
   A. All parts
II. **Symptoms (some or all may be present)**
   A. Digestive upset
   B. Heart failure
   C. Excitement or depression
   D. Oral irritation
   E. Decreased body temperature
III. **First Aid**
   A. If your dog is alert, induce vomiting.
   B. Call your veterinarian immediately.
   C. Observe for symptoms.

ONION (Allium)

I.   **Toxic Portion of Plant**

     A.   All parts

II.   **Symptoms (one or both may be present)**

     A.   Digestive upset

     B.   Weakness from hemolytic anemia

III. **First Aid**

     A.   If your dog is alert, induce vomiting.

     B.   Call your veterinarian immediately.

     C.   Observe for symptoms.

PANDA (Philodendron panduraeformae)

See Philodendron on page 224.

PEA (Lathyrus)

I.   **Toxic Portion of Plant**

     A.   All parts

     B.   Seeds especially

II.   **Symptoms (some or all may be present)**

     A.   Seizures

     B.   Paralysis

     C.   Depressed breathing

III. **First Aid**

     A.   If your dog is alert, induce vomiting.

     B.   Call your veterinarian immediately.

     C.   Observe for symptoms.

PEACE LILY (Spathiphyllum)

See Philodendron on page 224.

PENCIL CACTUS (Euphorbia tirucalli)

I. **Toxic Portion of Plant**

    A.   All parts

II. **Symptoms (one or both may be present)**

    A.   Digestive upset

    B.   Irritation of skin/blistering

III. **First Aid**

    A.   If your dog is alert, induce vomiting.

    B.   Call your veterinarian immediately.

    C.   Observe for symptoms.

PEONY (Paeonia)

I. **Toxic Portion of Plant**

    A.   Flowers

    B.   Seeds

II. **Symptoms (some or all may be present)**

    A.   Digestive upset

    B.   Central nervous system signs - tremors, seizures, staggering, loss of coordination, etc.

    C.   Depression

    D.   Collapse

    E.   Heart failure

    F.   Possible death

III. **First Aid**

    A.   If your dog is alert, induce vomiting.

    B.   Call your veterinarian immediately.

    C.   Observe for symptoms.

PHILODENDRON

I. **Toxic Portion of Plant**

    A.   All parts

II. **Symptoms (some or all may be present)**

A. Digestive upset
B. Irritation of mouth with possible swelling of the throat
C. Possible asphyxiation
D. Central nervous system signs - tremors, seizures, staggering, loss of coordination, etc.
E. Possible death

III. First Aid
A. If your dog is alert, induce vomiting.
B. Call your veterinarian immediately.
C. Observe for symptoms.

PLUMOSA FERN

See Asparagus Fern on page 235.

POINSETTIA (Euphorbia pulcherrima)

I. Toxic Portion of Plant
A. All parts

II. Symptoms (one or both may be present)
A. Digestive upset
B. Irritation to the mouth and stomach

III. First Aid
A. If your dog is alert, induce vomiting.
B. Call your veterinarian immediately.
C. Observe for symptoms.

POKEWEED (Phytolacca)

I. Toxic Portion of Plant
A. Roots

II. Symptoms (some or all may be present)
A. Digestive upset
B. Depression

C. Exhaustion

D. Coma

E. Possible death

III. First Aid

A. If your dog is alert, induce vomiting.

B. Call your veterinarian immediately.

C. Observe for symptoms.

POTATO

I. Toxic Portion of Plant

A. Leaves

B. Stems

C. Stalks

D. Sprouts

E. Tuber is edible.

II. Symptoms (some or all may be present)

A. Digestive upset

B. Heart failure

C. Depression/drowsiness

D. Drooling

E. Dilated pupils

III. First Aid

A. If your dog is alert, induce vomiting.

B. Call your veterinarian immediately.

C. Observe for symptoms.

POTHOS (Scindapsus)

See Philodendron on page 224.

PRECATORY BEAN (Abrus precatorius)

I. Toxic Portion of Plant

A. Beans are very poisonous.

II. **Symptoms (some or all may be present)**

A. Digestive upset

B. Fever

C. Staggering

D. Death

III. **First Aid**

A. If your dog is alert, induce vomiting.

B. Call your veterinarian immediately.

C. Observe for symptoms.

PRIMROSE (Primula)

I. **Toxic Portion of Plant**

A. All parts

II. **Symptom**

A. Digestive upset

III. **First Aid**

A. If your dog is alert, induce vomiting.

B. Call your veterinarian immediately.

C. Observe for symptoms.

PRIVET

I. **Toxic Portion of Plant**

A. Berries

B. Leaves

II. **Symptoms (one or both may be present)**

A. Digestive upset

B. Kidney damage

III. **First Aid**

A. If your dog is alert, induce vomiting.

B. Call your veterinarian immediately.

C. Observe for symptoms.

RAYLESS GOLDENROD

I. Toxic Portion of Plant

    A.   All parts

II. Symptoms (some or all may be present)

    A.   Digestive upset

    B.   Weakness

    C.   Constipation

    D.   Seizures

    E.   Liver damage/failure

    F.   Kidney damage

III. First Aid

    A.   If your dog is alert, induce vomiting.

    B.   Call your veterinarian immediately.

    C.   Observe for symptoms.

RED EMERALD (Philodendron Red Emerald)

See Philodendron on page 224.

RED-MARGINED DRACAENA (Dracaena marginata)

See Corn Plant on page 197.

RED PRINCESS (Philodendron Red Princess)

See Philodendron on page 224.

RHODODENDRON

See Azalea on page 189.

RIBBON PLANT (Dracaena sanderiana)

See Corn Plant on page 197.

SAGO PALM (Cycas)

See Cycad on page 200.

SCHEFFLERA (Brassaia actinophylla)

See Philodendron on page 224.

SNOW-ON-THE-MOUNTAIN (Euphorbia marginata)

I. **Toxic Portion of Plant**
   A. All parts
   B. Seeds are especially toxic.
   C. One leaf or seed may be deadly.

II. **Symptoms (some or all may be present)**
   A. Digestive upset
   B. Liver and kidney damage
   C. Central nervous system signs - tremors, seizures, staggering, loss of coordination, etc.
   D. Possible death

III. **First Aid**
   A. If your dog is alert, induce vomiting.
   B. Call your veterinarian immediately.
   C. Observe for symptoms.

STAR-OF-BETHLEHEM

I. **Toxic Portion of Plant**
   A. Bulb is most toxic.

II. **Symptoms (some or all may be present)**

A. Digestive upset
B. Excitement followed by depression, then coma
C. Possible death

III. First Aid
A. If your dog is alert, induce vomiting.
B. Call your veterinarian immediately.
C. Observe for symptoms.

STRING OF PEARLS/BEADS (Senecio rowleyanus)

I. Toxic Portion of Plant
A. All parts

II. Symptoms (one or both may be present)
A. Digestive upset
B. Irregular heartbeat

III. First Aid
A. If your dog is alert, induce vomiting.
B. Call your veterinarian immediately.
C. Observe for symptoms.

STRIPED DRACAENA (Dracaena deremensis Warnickei)

See Corn Plant on page 197.

SWEETHEART IVY (Hedera helix sweetheart)

See English Ivy on page 204.

TARO

See Elephant's Ear on page 204.

TARO VINE (Scindapsus aureus)

See Philodendron on page 224.

TAXUS (Yew)

I. **Toxic Portion of Plant**

    A.   All parts

    B.   Especially berries

II. **Symptoms (some or all may be present)**

    A.   Digestive upset

    B.   Excitement or depression

    C.   Heart failure

III. **First Aid**

    A.   If your dog is alert, induce vomiting.

    B.   Call your veterinarian immediately.

    C.   Observe for symptoms.

TOADSTOOLS

I. **Toxicity**

    A.   Many species of toadstools and mushrooms are poisonous, especially the Amanita species.

II. **Symptoms (some or all may be present)**

    A.   Digestive upset

    B.   Drooling

    C.   Constricted or dilated pupils

    D.   Shaking/shivering/muscle spasms

    E.   Weakness

    F.   Irregular heartbeat

    G.   Liver damage

    H.   Possible blood in urine

    I.   Possible coma and death

III. **First Aid**

    A.   If the dog is alert, induce vomiting and call a veterinarian.

B.   Identify the toadstool the dog has ingested. If the toadstool cannot be identified, obtain a sample of the fungus. Plants can be identified by veterinarians and by plant identification books.

C.   Observe for symptoms.

TOMATO (Lycopersicon)

I.   **Toxic Portion of Plant**
  A.   Leaves
  B.   Stems
  C.   Stalks
  D.   Fruit is edible.

II. **Symptoms (some or all may be present)**
  A.   Digestive upset
  B.   Depression/drowsiness
  C.   Drooling
  D.   Dilated pupils
  E.   Heart failure

III. **First Aid**
  A.   If your dog is alert, induce vomiting.
  B.   Call your veterinarian immediately.
  C.   Observe for symptoms.

VARIABLE DIEFFENBACHIA (Dieffenbachia picta)

See Dumb Cane on page 202.

VARIEGATED RUBBER PLANT (Ficus elastica variegata)

See Fiddle-leaf Fig on page 205.

WATER HEMLOCK (Cicuta)

I.   **Toxic Portion of Plant**
A.   Tuber mostly
II. **Symptoms (one or both may be present)**
A.   Central nervous system signs - tremors, seizures, staggering, loss of coordination, etc.
B.   Seizures
III. **First Aid**
A.   If your dog is alert, induce vomiting.
B.   Call your veterinarian immediately.
C.   Observe for symptoms.

WEEPING FIG (Ficus benjamina)

See Fiddle-leaf Fig on page 205.

WILD ACONITE

I.   **Toxic Portion of Plant**
A.   All parts
II. **Symptoms (some or all may be present)**
A.   Digestive upset with bloody diarrhea
B.   Disorientation
C.   Staggering
D.   Difficulty breathing
E.   Seizures
F.   Coma and possible death
III. **First Aid**
A.   If your dog is alert, induce vomiting.
B.   Call your veterinarian immediately.
C.   Observe for symptoms.

WISTERIA

I. **Toxic Portion of Plant**
   A.   All parts
II. **Symptom**
   A.   Digestive upset
III. **First Aid**
   A.   If your dog is alert, induce vomiting.
   B.   Call your veterinarian immediately.
   C.   Observe for symptoms.

YEW (Taxus)

See Japanese Yew on page 211 or Taxus on page 231.

PLANTS THAT CAUSE SKIN IRRITATION

There are two types of skin irritation caused by plants. The first is irritation caused by a reaction to the chemicals in the plant (usually in the plant's sap or resin). Examples include asparagus fern, chrysanthemum resin, manchineel sap, poinsettia sap and primrose leaves. The second type of skin irritation occurs from certain types of grasses (e.g., foxtail/grass awns) when tiny parts of the plant (spikelets) become embedded in and under the dog's skin (e.g., in the ears or in the webbing of the feet). If the plant spikelets are not removed, they may cause abscesses (i.e., infections). Your veterinarian may need to sedate your dog in order to remove the spikelets.

I. **List of Plants**

A. Asparagus fern

B. Chrysanthemum resin

C. Manchineel sap

D. Poinsettia sap

E. Primrose leaves

F. Foxtail/grass awns

II. **First Aid**

A. For everything except foxtail/grass awns, wash affected area with soap and water and cleanse with alcohol.

B. For foxtail/grass awns:

(1) Apply antibiotic ointment (e.g., Polysporin®) to the affected area.

(2) If the dog persistently licks or scratches the affected area, apply an Elizabethan collar.

(3) Contact your veterinarian for removal of spikelets or for more information.

NONPOISONOUS PLANTS

I. Warning

A. Even though many plants are not toxic, when ingested in quantity they can cause digestive upset. Also, even plants that are generally not considered to be poisonous can cause an allergic reaction that may be serious. Each dog is unique, and a plant that may cause no difficulties for one dog may be toxic for another.

II. Special Considerations

A. Plants may be sprayed with chemicals which can be toxic to dogs.

B. Often a dog will eat plants, especially grass, when the dog feels ill from something else. Grass, although not harmful, usually causes the dog to vomit. If your dog is eating plants or grass, observe for other signs of illness, and consult your veterinarian.

PART 6

—

OTHER POISONS

ACETAMINOPHEN (TYLENOL®) TOXICITY

Like many human drugs, Tylenol® is toxic to dogs. In fact, ingestion may be lethal if the dog does not receive veterinary treatment. No medications of any kind should be given to a dog without instructions from a veterinarian. And because dogs are curious by nature, all drugs should be kept out of your dog's reach to prevent accidental ingestion.

I. **Symptoms**
A. Listlessness
B. Difficulty breathing
C. Vomiting and/or diarrhea
D. Dark-colored urine

II. **First-Aid Materials**
A. Hydrogen peroxide
B. Eyedropper or dosage syringe

III. **First Aid**
A. If the pet is conscious, induce vomiting immediately by feeding the dog 1 teaspoon of hydrogen peroxide (mixed with 1 teaspoon milk if available). If the dog will not drink the mixture or if there is no milk available, then force-feed the dog the hydrogen peroxide using an eyedropper. If vomiting does not occur within 10 minutes, repeat the procedure twice.
B. Contact a veterinarian for further treatment regardless of whether you are successful at inducing vomiting.

ACIDS AND ALKALIS

Acids and alkalis can be found in a wide variety of products. Acids include: sulfuric (found in auto batteries and metal cleaners and polishes), hydrochloric (in metal cleaners and polishes), nitric (in permanent wave neutralizer), oxalic (in cleaning solutions, bleach, and furniture and floor polishes and waxes), carbolic acid or phenol (in antiseptics and disinfectants). Alkalis include: sodium hydroxide/lye (in aquarium products, drain cleaners and small batteries), potassium hydroxide (in cuticle remover and some small batteries), sodium phosphate (in abrasive cleaners), sodium carbonate (in dye removers and dishwasher soap). In addition, there are milder alkalis found in ammonia and bleaches. Ingestion of acids or alkalis can cause severe internal irritation as well as external burns. Because these poisons are extreme irritants, **do not induce vomiting**.

I. **Symptoms**
A. Salivating
B. Vomiting
C. Diarrhea
D. Weakness

II. **First-Aid Materials**
A. Milk of Magnesia®
B. Lemon juice
C. Vinegar
D. Baking soda
E. Eyedropper or dosage syringe

III. **First Aid**
A. **Do not induce vomiting**.
B. **For acid ingestion**, feed your dog 1 tablespoon Milk of Magnesia® using an eyedropper or dosage syringe.
C. **For acid burns**, flush areas with copious amounts of water. Apply a paste of 1 part baking soda to 2 parts water to burns.

D. **For alkali ingestion,**
   (1) Mix 1 teaspoon vinegar with 4 teaspoons water and feed the mixture to your dog using an eyedropper or dosage syringe, **or**
   (2) Feed your dog 1 tablespoon lemon juice using an eyedropper or dosage syringe. (You may mix 1 teaspoon of sugar into the lemon juice so that the dog will like it better.)
E. **For alkali burns,** flush the areas with copious amounts of water. Apply a solution of 1 cup vinegar to 4 cups water over areas.
F. Contact a veterinarian for additional instructions.

ANTIFREEZE TOXICITY

Antifreeze is a common poison to pets for three reasons: it is a commonly-used product, it is often improperly discarded, and it is sweet to the taste.

Antifreeze contains ethylene glycol which, when metabolized, causes kidney damage that is usually fatal. Even a small amount will cause severe illness or death. Because the toxin is rapidly absorbed, symptoms may appear as early as one hour after ingestion. Symptoms are vague and mimic those of many other conditions and diseases.

I. **Symptoms (some or all may be present)**
A. Increased thirst
B. Vomiting and diarrhea
C. Depression
D. Loss of coordination
E. The pet may show slight improvement in its condition before its kidneys fail.

II. **First-Aid Materials**
A. Hydrogen peroxide
B. Liquor (e.g., vodka, whiskey, gin, rum)
C. Eyedropper or dosage syringe

III. **First Aid**
A. If an exposure is suspected, induce vomiting by feeding the dog 1 teaspoon of hydrogen peroxide (mixed with 1 teaspoon milk if available). If the dog will not drink the mixture or if there is no milk available, then force-feed the dog the hydrogen peroxide using an eyedropper or dosage syringe. If vomiting does not occur within 10 minutes, repeat the procedure up to two times.
B. Get immediate veterinary help.
C. If a veterinarian cannot be found, then when vomiting ceases or

if vomiting cannot be induced, feed the dog using an eyedropper or dosage syringe 2 tablespoons of liquor (e.g., vodka, whiskey, gin, rum) mixed with 2 tablespoons of half and half cream. (If half and half cream is not available, then use milk or water.) Wait 10 minutes, and if there are no signs of depression or intoxication, administer another 1 tablespoon of liquor mixed with 1 tablespoon of half and half cream. (The ethanol in liquor competes with the ethylene glycol metabolism decreasing the amounts that may cause damage to the kidneys. It also promotes increased urination to allow faster excretion of the poison.)

D. Seek veterinary attention for further treatment.

ARSENIC POISONING

Arsenic poisoning can occur in dogs that ingest water or plants that have been contaminated with herbicides or pesticides containing arsenic. If your dog does ingest arsenic, early treatment is essential because arsenic is extremely toxic.

I.   **Symptoms (some or all may be present)**
A.   Abdominal pain
B.   Weakness
C.   Salivating
D.   Vomiting
E.   Diarrhea
F.   Shaking
G.   Staggering
H.   Collapse
I.   Death

II. **First-Aid Materials**
A.   Hydrogen peroxide
B.   Eyedropper or dosage syringe
C.   Raw egg whites

III. **First Aid**
A.   If an exposure is suspected, induce vomiting by feeding the dog 1 teaspoon of hydrogen peroxide (mixed with 1 teaspoon milk if available). If the dog will not drink the mixture or if there is no milk available, then force-feed the dog the hydrogen peroxide using an eyedropper or dosage syringe. If vomiting does not occur within 10 minutes, repeat the procedure up to two times.
B.   Get immediate veterinary help.
C.   If a veterinarian cannot be found, then when vomiting ceases or if vomiting cannot be induced, using an eyedropper slowly feed the dog 2 tablespoons of raw egg whites.

CHOCOLATE TOXICITY

Chocolate contains a substance called theobromine which cannot be readily metabolized by dogs. Even in small quantities, chocolate may be toxic to your dog.

I. **Symptoms (some or all may be present)**
A. Moderate to severe vomiting and diarrhea
B. Excitability and nervousness
C. Muscle tremors and/or seizures
D. Heart failure

II. **First-Aid Materials**
A. Hydrogen peroxide
B. Eyedropper or dosage syringe

III. **First Aid**
A. If the ingestion has occurred within the previous 6 hours, immediately induce vomiting by feeding the dog 1 teaspoon of hydrogen peroxide (mixed with 1 teaspoon milk if available). If the dog will not drink the mixture or if there is no milk available, then force-feed the dog the hydrogen peroxide using an eyedropper. If vomiting does not occur within 10 minutes, repeat the procedure twice.
B. See a veterinarian for further monitoring and supportive care.

ETHYLENE GLYCOL TOXICITY

Ethylene glycol is a chemical found in automobile antifreeze. Unfortunately, dogs find that antifreeze has a pleasant taste, and dogs that are outdoors unattended are therefore highly susceptible to ethylene glycol poisoning. When ethylene glycol is metabolized, it causes kidney damage that is usually fatal. Even a small amount will cause severe illness or death. Because the toxin is rapidly absorbed, symptoms may appear as early as one hour after ingestion. Symptoms are vague and mimic those of many other conditions and diseases.

I. **Symptoms (some or all may be present)**

A. Increased thirst

B. Vomiting and diarrhea

C. Depression

D. Loss of coordination

E. The pet may show slight improvement in its condition before its kidneys fail.

II. **First-Aid Materials**

A. Hydrogen peroxide

B. Liquor (e.g., vodka, whiskey, gin, rum)

C. Eyedropper or dosage syringe

III. **First Aid**

A. If an exposure is suspected, induce vomiting by feeding the dog 1 teaspoon of hydrogen peroxide (mixed with 1 teaspoon milk if available). If the dog will not drink the mixture or if there is no milk available, then force-feed the dog the hydrogen peroxide using an eyedropper or dosage syringe. If vomiting does not occur within 10 minutes, repeat the procedure up to two times.

B. Get immediate veterinary help.

C. If a veterinarian cannot be found, then when vomiting ceases or if vomiting cannot be induced, feed the dog using an eyedropper or dosage syringe 2 tablespoons of liquor (e.g., vodka, whiskey, gin, rum) mixed with 2 tablespoons of half and half cream. (If half and half cream is not available, then use milk or water.) Wait 10 minutes, and if there are no signs of depression or intoxication, administer another 1 tablespoon of liquor mixed with 1 tablespoon of half and half cream. (The ethanol in liquor competes with the ethylene glycol metabolism decreasing the amounts that may cause damage to the kidneys. It also promotes increased urination to allow faster excretion of the poison.)

D. Seek veterinary attention for further treatment.

FLEA PRODUCT TOXICITY

Flea products are chemicals, and sometimes dogs have reactions to them. It is important to follow the flea-product directions to minimize the risk to your dog. The relatively small risk associated with using flea products is justified, however, because fleas can spread parasites and infections, and they can cause fatal anemia.

I. **Symptoms**

A. Drooling longer than 20 minutes

B. Loss of appetite

C. Digestive upset

D. Seizures or muscle tremors (in severe cases)

E. Disorientation

II. **First-Aid Materials**

A. Shampoo that does not contain flea chemicals

III. **First Aid**

A. If chemicals have been applied to the dog, immediately wash off the product using shampoo and water. Repeat once.

B. See a veterinarian for an antidote, further monitoring, and supportive care.

IBUPROFEN TOXICITY

Ibuprofen (e.g., Advil®)is an anti-inflammatory drug that, for dogs, is very toxic. Because ibuprofen is a common household medication, dogs often have easy access to the drug. Some ibuprofen brands are sugar-coated and appeal to dogs. Human medications should never be given to pets without the advice of a veterinarian.

I. **Symptoms (some or all may be present)**

A. Digestive upset

B. Bloody stool

C. Depression

D. Staggering

E. Increased thirst

F. Increased frequency of urination

G. Liver disease

H. Kidney disease

I. Seizures

II. **First-Aid Materials**

A. Hydrogen peroxide

B. Eyedropper or dosage syringe

III. **First Aid**

A. If the pet is conscious, induce vomiting immediately by feeding the dog 1 teaspoon of hydrogen peroxide (mixed with 1 teaspoon of milk if available). If the dog will not drink the mixture or if there is no milk available, then force-feed the dog the hydrogen peroxide using an eyedropper or dosage syringe. If vomiting does not occur within 10 minutes, repeat the procedure twice.

B. Contact your veterinarian for further treatment regardless of whether you have been successful at inducing vomiting.

LEAD TOXICITY

Lead poisoning is becoming less common because of an increased awareness of its health hazards. Lead poisoning is seen more commonly in dogs than in cats because dogs tend to chew extraneous objects to a greater extent than do cats. Products like paint, plaster, caulking, linoleum, solder, improperly glazed dishes, fishing sinkers and golf balls sometimes contain lead.

I. Symptoms
A. Digestive upset
B. Loss of appetite
C. Personality/behavior change
D. Seizures and blindness (in severe cases)

II. First-Aid Materials
A. Hydrogen peroxide
B. Eyedropper
C. Raw egg white

III. First Aid
A. If the ingestion has occurred within the last 6 hours, immediately induce vomiting by feeding the dog 1 teaspoon of hydrogen peroxide (mixed with 1 teaspoon milk if available). If the dog will not drink the mixture or if there is no milk available, then force-feed the dog the hydrogen peroxide using an eyedropper. If vomiting does not occur within 10 minutes, repeat the procedure twice.
B. After vomiting has stopped, or if you are unsuccessful at inducing vomiting, mix 1 raw egg white with 2 cups of water. Encourage the dog to drink as much of this solution as possible, or slowly administer 1/2 cup (for small dogs) up to 2 cups (for a large dog) with an eyedropper or dosage syringe.
C. See a veterinarian for further monitoring and supportive care.

PETROLEUM DISTILLATES

Petroleum distillates include gasoline, kerosene, paint thinner, lighter fluid, mineral spirits, diesel fuel, some household all-purpose lubricating oils (e.g., WD-40® and 3-IN-ONE® household oil) and petroleum-based insecticides (e.g., Raid®). Some furniture polishes and cleaners also contain petroleum distillates. If ingestion of petroleum distillates does occur, **do not induce vomiting.** Vomiting may cause the petroleum to become aspirated (i.e., breathed into the lungs), which will cause respiratory irritations and possibly pneumonia.

I.   Symptoms (some or all may be present)

A.   Salivation

B.   Odor of petroleum

C.   Difficulty breathing

II.   First-Aid Materials

A.   Any vegetable oil

B.   Eyedropper or dosage syringe

III. First Aid

A.   Feed the dog 1-2 tablespoons of vegetable oil using an eyedropper or dosage syringe.

B.   Contact a veterinarian immediately.

RAT POISON

Rat poisons are laced in a grain base which intrigues dogs. When a dog eats rat poison, the poison interferes with the dog's ability to make vitamin K. Vitamin K is essential in causing blood to clot, and without the vitamin, a dog will hemorrhage internally. Because the symptoms from rat poison take several days to appear, early treatment is essential if an exposure is even suspected.

I. Symptoms (some or all may be present)

A. None for several days

B. Weakness – frequently the first symptom

C. Pale, white or bruised gums

D. Bruises on the dog's body

E. Bloody urine and/or stools

F. Blue-green feces or vomitus – some rat baits contain a blue-green dye

G. Death – may occur within 24 hours of first symptoms

II. First-Aid Materials

A. Hydrogen peroxide

B. Eyedropper or dosage syringe

III. First Aid

A. If exposure has occurred within 6 hours, immediately induce vomiting by feeding the dog 1 teaspoon of hydrogen peroxide (mixed with 1 teaspoon of milk if available). If the dog will not drink the mixture or if there is no milk available, then force-feed the dog the hydrogen peroxide using an eyedropper or dosage syringe. If vomiting does not occur within 10 minutes, repeat the procedure twice.

B. Regardless of whether you have been able to induce vomiting, seek veterinary care immediately. Your veterinarian will prescribe vitamin K as an antidote and may also prescribe medicines to slow absorption of the poison.

SNAIL BAIT

Snail bait is poisonous to pets because it contains the chemical metaldehyde. This product, like rat poison, is made with a tasty base that attracts not only snails but also dogs.

I. Symptoms

A. Loss of coordination

B. Muscle tremors or convulsions

C. Increased heart rate

II. First-Aid Materials

A. Hydrogen peroxide

B. Eyedropper or dosage syringe

III. First Aid

A. Induce vomiting if exposure is suspected. (Do not attempt to induce vomiting if the pet exhibits any loss of coordination or is having a seizure because the pet could aspirate vomit into its lungs.) Induce vomiting by feeding the dog 1 teaspoon of hydrogen peroxide (mixed with 1 teaspoon of milk if available). If the dog will not drink the mixture or if there is no milk available, then force-feed the dog the hydrogen peroxide using an eyedropper or dosage syringe. If vomiting does not occur within 10 minutes, repeat the procedure twice.

B. Contact a veterinarian immediately.

STRYCHNINE POISONING

Strychnine is sometimes an ingredient in products sold to kill insects and rodents. The products are laced with a sweetener to attract the animal and generally contain enough strychnine that even ingestion of a small amount of the product will kill the pest. Unfortunately, strychnine is highly poisonous, and even a small amount will likely kill your dog. If your dog does ingest strychnine, immediate action is necessary.

I. Symptoms

A. Symptoms may appear within 2 hours of ingestion.

B. The dog may appear to be apprehensive or nervous.

C. Stiffness may develop, leading to severe seizures. These seizures can be provoked or exacerbated by external stimuli (e.g., noise, trauma, etc.).

D. Exhaustion and death may shortly follow the onset of symptoms.

II. First-Aid Materials

A. Hydrogen peroxide

B. Eyedropper or dosage syringe

III. First Aid

A. If the pet is conscious and alert, immediately induce vomiting by feeding the dog 1 teaspoon of hydrogen peroxide (mixed with 1 teaspoon of milk if available). If the dog will not drink the mixture or if there is no milk available, then force-feed the dog the hydrogen peroxide using an eyedropper or dosage syringe. If vomiting does not occur within 10 minutes, repeat the procedure twice.

B. To keep your dog from injuring itself during a seizure, block off access to stairways and move any objects or furniture that may cause injury. If a seizure does occur, see page 122 for additional instructions.

C. Keep the dog in a quiet environment.

D. Seek veterinary help.

YARD CHEMICALS

A variety of chemicals in fertilizers and pesticides can cause illness either from inhalation, contact or ingestion. Symptoms of illness may be delayed for days, but may be quite severe. Avoid exposing your dog to these toxins by keeping your dog indoors during and immediately after yard fertilization and spraying, and if you are using an insecticide indoors, keep your dog out of the room until the chemicals have dissipated. Never spray your dog with an insecticide that is not labeled specifically for use on dogs.

I. Symptoms (some or all may be present)

A. Listlessness

B. Loss of appetite

C. Difficulty breathing

D. Vomiting

E. Diarrhea

F. Skin irritation from contact (typically the pads of the feet)

II. First Aid Materials

A. Shampoo

III. First Aid

A. If the dog gets chemicals on its fur, bathe the dog with dog shampoo (or any mild moisturizing shampoo if dog shampoo is not available). While restraining the dog, apply the shampoo and let it stand for 10 minutes before rinsing well.

B. Seek veterinary assistance for additional advice and treatment.

PART 7

—

DISEASES THAT CAN
BECOME EMERGENCIES

GENERAL INFORMATION

There are many diseases and conditions that are not emergencies but can develop into emergencies if untreated. All of the diseases and conditions discussed in Part 7 of this book call for veterinarian care to prevent a crisis from developing. Early treatment may result in complete cure, whereas lack of proper care can eventually lead to a crisis and possibly death.

Because your dog is unable to communicate effectively when there is a problem developing, always try to be aware of any changes in your dog's behavior, appearance or physical condition. If your dog has any history of any diseases or conditions that may become an emergency, ask your veterinarian for signs to look for that may indicate a return or worsening of the situation. If in doubt, always seek veterinary advice early rather than waiting until a more serious situation develops.

For additional information on prevention of emergencies see the chapter starting on page 12 and the Appendix on page 288.

DENTAL DISEASE

Dental-related emergencies can be avoided by providing your dog with regular veterinary dental care. A dog's teeth should be checked by a veterinarian for dental disease at least every six months. Dental disease can cause pain, discomfort, and infection in the dog's mouth, and if left untreated, it can be life-threatening. Any infection in the mouth can spread into the bloodstream where it can cause a variety of problems, including damage to the heart, liver and kidneys.

I. Symptoms of dental disease (some or all may be present)
A. Bad breath
B. Difficulty chewing
C. Brownish-yellow-green plaque buildup on teeth
D. Recessed, reddened gums
E. Sneezing
F. Swelling below eyes
G. Drooling

II. Home care
A. Check the dog's teeth at home once weekly by pulling back the corner of the dog's lips. Look for recessed, reddened gums and brownish-yellow-green plaque buildup on teeth.
B. Brush a dog's teeth using pet toothpaste and a finger toothbrush two to five times weekly or apply a pet dental hygiene spray with a cotton ball to slow development of dental problems.

III. Veterinary care
A. The dog's teeth should be checked for dental disease at least twice each year by a veterinarian.
B. Treatment or extraction of diseased teeth may be necessary.

INFECTIONS AND FEVER

Infections and fever are unpredictable when left unattended. Many mild infections and fevers may resolve on their own; however, some can be overwhelming and cause long-term complications or death. Even a simple ear infection can be serious.

I. **Symptoms of Infections and Fever (some or all may be present)**
A. Pain and swelling at site of infection
B. Elevated temperature
C. Listlessness
D. Other general signs of illness such as vomiting, diarrhea, coughing, sneezing, and loss of appetite

II. **Home Care**
A. Use all medications as prescribed by the veterinarian.
B. Do not deviate from the dosage or the time interval on the label.
C. Use all antibiotics until gone, unless directed otherwise. Sporadic use of antibiotics can cause bacteria to become resistant to treatment.
D. Take the dog's temperature daily to monitor progress. See page 38.

III. **Veterinarian Care**
A. When you suspect that your dog has an infection, contact your veterinarian immediately; antibiotics may be necessary.
B. If the dog's condition does not improve, or worsens, while on medication, again contact your veterinarian. It may be necessary to change medications or to perform a culture to further identify the problem.

CANCERS

Certain types of cancers progress slowly and cause only minimal discomfort in their early stages. Dogs that have these types of cancers may lead a contented lifestyle for some time. Over time, however, a dog with any cancer is likely to develop complications that may be life-threatening if not tended to promptly. By tending to these problems, you may enable your pet to be comfortable and enjoy a longer life. For example, if a dog suffers from weight loss or a decrease in appetite from the disease, the dog's diet can be adjusted by your veterinarian to provide more nutrition in smaller quantities.

I. Home Care

A. Loss or decrease in appetite is one of the most common side effects of cancer. Dogs can be encouraged to eat by warming their food, hand feeding them, placing their food on a platter instead of in a bowl, and arranging the food in small portions on the platter. If all else fails, try changing the type of food.

B. Avoid stressing pets that have chronic disease.

C. Increase access to water by placing several water bowls throughout the house and where the dog lies.

D. Help your dog out to the bathroom at least four times per day.

E. Notify your veterinarian of any change in appetite.

F. Keep the dog clean and dry.

G. When a problem arises, contact your veterinarian immediately.

II. Veterinary Care

A. The veterinarian can recommend ways to help keep your dog comfortable.

B. Medications can be used to prevent further complications.

C. A complete physical examination may indicate that surgery may be necessary to prolong the dog's life and provide comfort.

D. Nutritional consultation and diet change may be recommended.

LONG-TERM ILLNESSES

Dogs that have chronic diseases, such as liver and kidney disorders, usually cope reasonably well with the problem. Chronic diseases occur gradually, enabling the dog to adjust to the change in organ function without suffering many side effects. With a chronic disease, eventually there will be enough loss in organ function that the dog's condition will begin to decline more quickly.

I. Home Care

A. Loss or decrease in appetite is one of the most common side effects of cancer. Techniques you may use to encourage your dog to eat include warming the dog's food, placing the food on a platter instead of in a bowl, and arranging the food in small portions on the platter rather than in one big clump. If all else fails, try hand feeding or try changing the type of food.

B. Avoid causing stress to pets with chronic disease.

C. Increase access to water by placing several water bowls throughout the house.

D. Help your dog out to the bathroom at least four times per day.

E. Notify your veterinarian of any change in appetite or behavior.

F. Keep the dog clean and dry.

G. When a problem arises with a chronically ill dog, contact a veterinarian immediately.

II. Veterinary Care

A. A veterinarian can recommend ways to help keep your dog comfortable.

B. Medications can be used to prevent further deterioration or lessen complications. For example, a potassium deficiency caused by kidney disease is easily treated with a supplement.

C. A complete physical examination may be necessary to determine the best treatment to prolong your dog's life and provide comfort.

D. Nutritional consultation and diet change may be recommended.

SKIN IRRITATIONS

Skin irritations may cause severe discomfort to your pet. In addition, complications can arise from skin conditions, including the spread of infection internally and dehydration (if large areas are affected).

I. Home Care

A. Skin conditions should be tended to immediately to prevent the condition from worsening.

B. Shampooing the pet will likely provide temporary relief from its symptoms. Use a shampoo for dogs (moisturizing shampoo is best). While restraining the dog, lather the pet and let stand for 15-20 minutes. Rinse well with warm tap water. Next, mix 1 tablespoon of bath oil (e.g., Alpha Keri®) with 2 quarts of warm tap water. Then pour the bath-oil mixture over the dog's coat, being careful not to get any in its eyes. Let the coat dry naturally. Consult your veterinarian for the proper type of shampoo and for specific instructions.

C. If the dog is biting itself, it may be necessary to apply an Elizabethan collar to prevent more damage to the skin. See page 48 on how to make and use an Elizabethan collar.

D. If your dog is biting and scratching itself, apply a wrap or an Elizabethan collar. (See pages 37 and 48 respectively.)

II. Veterinary Care

A. Untreated skin conditions may lead to serious complications. Medications are available to alleviate skin irritations and hasten healing.

B. Your veterinarian can also determine if your dog's skin condition is one that could be contagious to humans.

SOFT STOOLS/DIARRHEA

Pets can have soft stools or diarrhea without showing other signs of illness. If this condition persists without treatment, the dog could suffer complications, including malnutrition from improper absorption of nutrients, dehydration, and anemia from slow loss of small quantities of blood from bowel irritation.

I.   Home Care

A.   If there is no vomiting, feed the dog Kaopectate® using an eyedropper or dosage syringe:

    (1) 1 to 2 teaspoons for dogs weighing less than 20 pounds,

    (2) 3 to 4 teaspoons for dogs weighing 20 or more pounds.

B.   Repeat Step A every 4 to 6 hours for adult dogs and every 2 to 4 hours for puppies less than 14 weeks old.

C.   Withhold food for 2-4 hours if diarrhea is present and if there is no other symptom of illness. Withhold both food and water if the dog is also vomiting, but do not withhold water for more than 2 hours. Do not withhold water if the dog is not vomiting. The time period for withholding food should be based on whether your pet is a normal, healthy adult versus a puppy, an elderly dog or a dog with any special or compromising conditions. If your dog has diabetes or any other type of illness or medical condition, consult your veterinarian first before withholding food and water.

D.   When you do resume feeding your dog, the best home remedy for diarrhea is to prepare a 50/50 mixture of boiled hamburger (drain off the water and fat) and plain cooked rice. Appropriate feedings are as follows:

    (1) 1/4 cup of the mixture 4 times per day for small dogs,

    (2) 1/2 cup of the mixture 4 times per day for medium dogs,

    (3) 3/4 cup of the mixture 4 times per day for large dogs.

Your veterinarian may wish to adjust the servings or may

recommend a prescription diet instead.

E. Note the frequency and substance of the diarrhea.

F. If symptoms persist for more than 4 hours, or if they worsen or return, contact the pet's doctor immediately.

G. If a dog has other signs along with the diarrhea (e.g., vomiting, loss of coordination, fatigue, etc.) contact a veterinarian.

H. Because some infections can be transmitted to people, wash your hands after handling the dog or cleaning up accidents.

II. Veterinary Care

A. Your veterinarian may request a stool sample for examination under the microscope (to check for intestinal parasites).

B. Proper diagnosis and medication from your veterinarian can prevent serious side effects from the diarrhea.

INTESTINAL PARASITES

Intestinal parasites, which include worms and protozoa, can cause serious illness if untreated. In general, most infestations are mild at first but then become serious as time progresses. If parasites are left untreated, fatal anemia from chronic blood loss and life-threatening malnutrition can develop. It is important to have a stool sample checked under the microscope for worm eggs. If any eggs are present, your veterinarian can prescribe the proper medication.

The most common parasites in dogs include roundworms, tapeworms, hookworms and whipworms. Protozoa infestations include coccidia, giardia and toxoplasmosis. Some of these infections can be spread to people.

I. Symptoms (some or all may be present)
A. Weight loss
B. Diarrhea or soft stools
C. Blood and/or mucus in stools
D. Listlessness
E. Vomiting
F. Dull hair coat
G. Pot-bellied appearance
H. Worms in the stool or under the dog's tail

II. Home prevention
A. Clean the yard of stools at least once per day.
B. Practice good flea control. Fleas spread one type of tapeworm.
C. Never feed a dog raw meat.
D. Provide clean, fresh water for your outdoor dog because outside water may contain infectious protozoa or bacteria.
E. If you see any worms in the stool, contact your veterinarian.
F. Avoid over-the-counter worm medications; they may not be the proper choice for your pet's illness.

III. Veterinary care
A. Have a stool specimen examined by a veterinarian at least twice per year.
B. Use worm medications as directed.

EXTERNAL PARASITES - FLEAS

External parasites include fleas, ticks and lice. These parasites not only cause blood loss (sometimes resulting in anemia) but may also transmit diseases. It is important to note that a severe flea infestation may be extremely difficult to treat effectively, both in terms of your pet and your home. Prevention (e.g., use of a flea collar, flea spray and/or flea pills) and early treatment are critical in keeping the situation from developing into a major problem.

Whenever you are using flea products either as prevention or treatment, it is important to read all instructions thoroughly. Products that are used improperly or used in the wrong combination can be harmful to your dog. If your dog has an adverse reaction to any type of flea treatment, discontinue the treatment and contact a veterinarian immediately.

I.   Symptoms (some or all may be present)

A.   Fleas visible crawling through the dog's hair coat or jumping on or off of the dog – They are very small dark insects, so small they are difficult to see. An enlarged illustration appears on page 267.

B.   Flea droppings – Even if you cannot see the fleas, you may see flea droppings, which appear as black specks throughout the dog's hair coat. These black specks are actually the fleas' waste products that consist of the dog's blood.

C.   Weakness from anemia

D.   Weight loss

E.   Scratching (though not all dogs with fleas will scratch)

II. Pet care

A.   Consult your veterinarian. A number of external parasite-control protocols can be prescribed.

B.   All products used should be labeled for dogs. These products should be used only as directed.

C. Bathe the pet in flea shampoo to remove the fleas and the flea droppings.

D. Treat the dog using a flea spray approved for use on dogs. The flea spray will kill residual fleas and keep other fleas off. Treat regularly with flea spray as directed by your veterinarian.

E. A veterinarian-prescribed flea collar may be used with the spray.

F. There are two types of flea pills available for your dog. One kills fleas that bite your dog, and the other prevents flea eggs from hatching. The type that kills fleas must be administered every three days, whereas the one that prevents fleas from hatching is taken only once per month. Also, the type that kills the fleas contains cythioate and may require additional precautions, especially if used in conjunction with other flea treatments.

G. Begin flea treatments as soon as you are aware of a flea problem. The longer you wait, the more difficult it will be to get rid of them.

H. If you witness any unusual reactions to any flea treatments (e.g., drooling lasting longer than 20 minutes, tremors, seizures, respiratory difficulty, etc.), discontinue the treatments immediately, and contact your veterinarian.

III. Environmental treatment

A. Inside the house:

(1) The dogs and the environment should be treated at the same time.

(2) Vacuum the home thoroughly.

(3) Discard vacuum cleaner bag.

(4) Wash the dog's bedding regularly.

(5) Using hand-held premises spray, treat all corners, baseboards, throw rugs, closets and cracks where foggers will not penetrate. Follow the instructions as directed on the product label.

(6) Place foggers strategically through the house in each closed room. Foggers will not penetrate through doorways or

down hallways. Follow the instructions on the label.

(7) Check environmental treatment inside the house two weeks after treatment by placing a pan of warm water on the floor before bedtime. Fleas are attracted to warmth and moisture, and if there are any remaining in your house, you should find some in the pan the next day.

(8) Repeat the above 7 steps in 2-4 weeks, if necessary.

B. Outside the house treatment:

(1) Treat the yard with a yard and kennel spray as directed on the product label.

(2) Keep outside rest areas clean and dry.

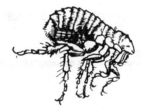

Flea

EXTERNAL PARASITES - LICE

External parasites include fleas, ticks and lice. These parasites not only cause blood loss, sometimes resulting in life-threatening anemia, but may also transmit diseases. Lice in large numbers can drain enough blood to kill a dog.

I. **General information**

A. Lice are slightly larger than fleas, and unlike fleas, their backs are flat. See illustration below.

B. The eggs or nits are seen as light specks along the hair shafts.

II. **Pet care**

A. Bathe your dog in a flea and tick shampoo as directed.

B. Once the dog is dry, apply a flea and tick spray approved for use on dogs.

C. Contact your family doctor and your veterinarian for details on transmission to people.

EXTERNAL PARASITES - TICKS

External parasites include fleas, ticks and lice. These parasites not only cause blood loss, sometimes resulting in life-threatening anemia, but may also transmit diseases. Ticks in large numbers can drain enough blood to kill a small dog.

I. **General Information**

A. Ticks are eight-legged parasites. See illustration on page 270.

B. The tick's body is flat, hard, and shiny but becomes soft and enlarged after feeding on a dog.

C. Ticks may carry diseases such as Lyme disease and Rocky Mountain spotted fever and tick paralysis.

D. Ticks embed their mouth parts only into the skin. It is not possible for a tick's head to get left behind in the dog's skin (i.e., when you remove the tick), but it is possible for the area to become infected or irritated mimicking the presence of something under the skin.

II. **How to remove a tick**

A. Apply a flea and tick spray for dogs directly on the tick, and wait one minute. Then, using tweezers or wearing disposable gloves, apply constant pull while grasping the tick's body. The tick should release.

B. Do not try to burn the tick or apply any other type of chemical to the tick. If flea or tick spray is not available, simply pull with constant pressure until the tick releases.

C. Dispose of the tick carefully. Make sure it is dead by spraying it with tick spray, or dispose of it by flushing it down the toilet. Avoid touching the tick with your bare hands.

D. Apply antibiotic ointment to the area where the tick was removed.

E.   If any unusual symptoms develop after the removal of the tick, contact your veterinarian.

III. Prevention

A.   Use a tick spray on a regular basis or use a flea and tick collar.
B.   Examine your dog every time the pet comes into the house from outside or at least once daily.

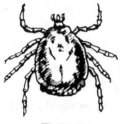

Tick

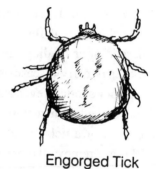

Engorged Tick

PART 8

—

MISCELLANEOUS

DELIVERIES

While most deliveries are routine and can be accomplished without any human intervention, sometimes complications occur. This chapter will assist you in identifying delivery problems.

I. **Preparation for Delivery**

A. Gather the following materials: a large box, clean towels, thread, warm water bottles and emergency formula. (See page 276 for a homemade emergency formula.)

B. Make sure the dog has a clean nesting area for the delivery. A large box 2 to 3 feet square and 6 inches high lined with a clean towel is ideal for a small dog, while a corner of a room or closet with a large clean towel or sheet is appropriate for large dogs.

C. Handle the dog as little as possible.

II. **Helping with a Delivery**

A. Try not to disturb the dog during the delivery process, but try to monitor her progress by quietly observing her actions.

B. If a puppy is being passed and is having difficulty clearing the vulva, you may exert gentle downward pressure on the puppy to help it pass.

C. If the mother is not cleaning the puppies after delivery, use a towel and remove any fluid from the nose and mouth. Then dry the puppy using a gentle rubbing action.

D. Occasionally the umbilical cord will not separate from the mother and puppy. If this occurs, take a thread and tie a knot 1/2 inch from the puppy's belly, and then cut the cord with scissors between the knot and the mother dog. This will prevent bleeding from tearing the cord. (See illustration on page 274.)

E. If a puppy is not breathing, continue to stimulate the puppy by rubbing it vigorously; at the same time blow into its nose every 5 seconds to give it air. Try this for at least 5 minutes.

F. The puppies should be placed at the mother's breast to ensure they nurse. Keep track of any puppies that do not nurse; they may need to be hand fed.

G. If the puppies cry, they may be hungry, cold, or sick. Contact your veterinarian if the crying persists.

III. Signs of a Difficult Delivery

A. If more than 20 minutes pass between puppies and the mother is having strong contractions, call your veterinarian.

B. If labor continues for more than an hour without the birth of a puppy, call your veterinarian.

C. When there is a weak contraction for a period of 1 hour between bouts of active labor, but no puppy is delivered, call your veterinarian.

D. If you observe any evidence of unusual pain during the delivery, such as crying or excessive biting or licking of the hind quarters, call your veterinarian.

E. If the pregnancy exceeds 70 days, call your veterinarian.

F. If there is an unusual discharge coming from the vulva under the tail, call your veterinarian. Normal discharge is green (not black, bloody, cloudy, or foul-smelling).

G. If there is normal greenish discharge without the birth of a puppy, call your veterinarian.

H. If the dog shows symptoms of illness, like depression, vomiting, diarrhea or weakness, call your veterinarian.

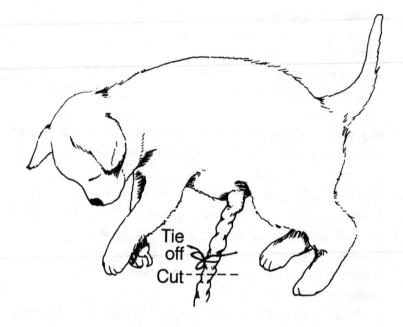

Tie
off
Cut

RAISING ORPHAN PUPPIES

When puppies have been abandoned or when the mother does not nurse her puppies, the puppies will need special care if they are to survive. Raising orphan puppies can be very rewarding but demands much time, motivation, and devotion. Unlike adult dogs, puppies have little body reserve and need highly regimented feeding and care schedules.

I. **Materials Needed**

A. Cotton balls

B. Light bulb or heat lamp

C. Pet nurser

D. Eyedropper

E. Formula

F. Scale for weighing

G. Thermometer

II. **Hygiene/Husbandry**

A. The puppy's nest area should be cleaned three times daily to prevent disease. Bed the area with newspaper or towels.

B. Store all formula as directed on the label to prevent spoilage.

C. Chilling is one of the leading causes of death among newborns. Keep the puppies warm with a heat lamp, heating pad, or hot water bottles. However, take care that the heat source is not too hot, and prepare a box that provides enough room for the puppies to move away from the heat source if they become too hot. Heating pads must be monitored closely to regulate temperature and prevent fire hazard. **Do not place a heating pad or hot water bottle on top of the puppies**.

D. The environmental temperature should be kept at 85-90 degrees from days 1-7. The temperature should be lowered to 80 degrees during week 2. Weeks 3-5, the temperature should be lowered to

75 degrees, then decreased again to 70 degrees at week 6.

E. Urinations and bowel movements must be stimulated after each meal. This is accomplished by moistening a cotton ball with warm water and gently wiping the puppy's bottom and abdomen.

F. Weigh each puppy and take its temperature daily.

III. Feeding

A. Use a pet nurser, if available, to feed the puppies. The hole in the nurser should leak milk slowly from the bottle without pressure. An eyedropper may be used temporarily if a nurser is unavailable.

B. Never feed a chilled puppy; make sure the orphan is warm prior to feeding.

C. Commercial formulas for newborns or infants are recommended over homemade diets. Homemade diets tend to lack balanced nutrition. If a commercial formula is not available, the following can be substituted temporarily:

EMERGENCY FORMULA RECIPE #1
8 oz. homogenized whole milk
1 teaspoon salad oil
2 egg yolks
1 drop infant vitamins

EMERGENCY FORMULA RECIPE # 2
1/3 cup nonfat dried milk
1/4 cup cottage cheese
1/8 cup corn oil
Add enough water to make 2 cups volume
Mix in blender

D. When using a commercially-available formula, follow the directions on the label regarding preparation, the frequency of feedings, and the amount to be fed. Whether you are using a commercial formula or a home preparation, it is important to note that the size, age and breed of the puppy will dictate what is appropriate in terms of feeding. Therefore, you should contact a veterinarian for advice specific to your puppy's needs. Until you are able to reach a veterinarian for professional advice, use the following guidelines for feeding:

(1) Amount of food per feeding based on size of puppy:
    (a) Puppies weighing 2 oz.: feed 1/2 teaspoon.
    (b) Puppies weighing 4 oz.: feed 1 teaspoon.
    (c) Puppies weighing 8 oz.: feed 2 teaspoons.
    (d) Puppies weighing 16 oz.: feed 4 teaspoons.

(2) Frequency of feeding based on age:
    (a) In the first week of life, feed every 2 to 4 hours.
    (b) In the second week of life, feed every 4 hours.
    (c) In the third week of life, feed every 6 hours.
    (d) In the fourth week of life, feed every 6 hours, and begin to mix the formula with canned puppy food. Offer these meals on a flat plate and allow the puppy to play in it to encourage self-feeding.

E. Urinations and bowel movements must be stimulated after each meal. This is accomplished by moistening a cotton ball with warm water and gently wiping the puppy's bottom and abdomen.

F. Overfeeding may cause diarrhea. Consult a veterinarian immediately if diarrhea occurs because puppies dehydrate easily.

IV. Signs of Illness

A. Crying (indicates that the puppies are either hungry, chilled, or sick)

B. Restlessness

C. Loss of appetite

D. Fever

E. Weight loss or lack of weight gain

F. Pot-bellied appearance

G. Vomiting or diarrhea

THE HOSPITALIZED DOG

When your pet must be hospitalized, you should make a list of questions for your veterinarian. In this chapter, a list of questions has been compiled for you, though you may wish to add more depending on the situation. If your dog does need hospitalization, don't simply ask the questions, but also write down the answers. If you make a written record of the answers, you will be better able to track your dog's progress based on the initial observations of the veterinarian.

I. Basic Guidelines

A. Leave a telephone number where someone can be reached at all times so that any changes in the dog's condition or treatment can be discussed.

B. Check with the doctors about their pet visitation policy.
Visitation is helpful not only to the pet but also for the owner.

C. If financial limits are affecting the care your dog may receive, inquire whether financial aid is available.

D. Determine how many progress reports will be shared during the day and whether you should call or they should call you.

II. Questions To Ask About the Problem

A. What is my dog's problem?

B. Does my pet have more than one problem, and, if so, are the problems related?

C. If there are several possible problems, are there tests to confirm the diagnosis?

III. Questions to Ask About Determining the Problem (Diagnosis)

A. What tests are available to diagnose my pet?

B. What information will the tests give?

C. Can the test results change the type of treatment my dog is receiving?

D. What is the cost of testing?

E. How invasive are the tests? How much pain will they cause and is there any risk associated with the tests?

IV. Questions To Ask About the Outcome (Prognosis)

A. What is my dog's prognosis?

B. Will this condition return?

C. Will this condition have any long-term side effects?

D. What is an average recovery time?

V. Questions To Ask About the Treatment

A. What will the treatment involve?

B. How much time will treatments take?

C. How expensive are the medications?

D. What side effects will be involved with the medicines?

E. If surgery is recommended:

    (1) Is there more than one procedure that can be done?

    (2) Is there a medical alternative to a surgical procedure?

    (3) How many of these surgeries do you perform per year?

    (4) Should I see a specialist?

F. What type of care will need to be provided after the dog returns home?

G. Are follow-up doctor visits recommended?

THE LOST DOG

One of the most frightening events for a dog owner is to lose a pet. Because of a dog's curiosity and instinct, it is often prone to roam. In particular, unaltered dogs have a high incidence of roaming because of urges to find a mate. Proper identification will improve your chances of recovering your lost dog. If your initial attempts to locate your pet are unsuccessful, do not give up hope; many animals return home days, weeks, or months later. Even with proper identification, the dog's chances of being found can be greatly increased by following the steps described below.

I. Information about the Lost Dog

A. List the dog's sex, breed, color, age, name and any distinguishing characteristics.

B. Make a list of several numbers (including the veterinarian's number) for people to call if the dog is found.

C. Find a picture of the dog, if possible.

D. Decide whether to offer a reward, and if so, what amount.

II. Daily Dog-Owner Efforts

A. Visit shelters daily to search for the dog.
(Do not assume someone will call if the pet arrives at the shelter. Most shelters deal with hundreds of pets each day. Daily visits are important because dogs are frequently euthanized after two days if not claimed or adopted.)

B. Contact all local veterinarians by phone about the missing dog.

C. Drive through local neighborhoods calling for and asking about the dog.

D. Have neighbors help in the search. Ask them to check their garages and storage sheds.

E. Post "Lost Dog" notices. See Appendix page 283.
(1) Include all identifying information. (See Section I above.)
(2) Include a picture.

280

(3) Indicate if there is a reward.

(4) Use waterproof ink and sturdy paper or poster board.

(5) Make the sign large so that it can be read from a distance.

(6) Post signs at all major intersections within at least a 3-mile radius of the dog's home.

(7) Post signs at local pet stores and other businesses (with their permission).

(8) Post signs at veterinary offices.

III. Organizations to Contact

A. Contact the local humane society.

(1) Ask whether they have your pet.

(2) Inquire about volunteers who run a lost and found or rescue service.

B. Contact other local shelters such as the dog/animal pound.

IV. Use of the Media

A. Run a classified advertisement for at least two weeks.

B. Check with radio and television; they often donate time during their news broadcasts to help find lost pets.

APPENDICES

LOST PET INFORMATION

Use the following form to help find a lost dog. Duplicate this form and post it according to the instructions found in the chapter The Lost Dog (starting on page 280).

LOST DOG

DESCRIPTION/BREED_____

COLOR(S)_____

SEX _____   AGE_____   WEIGHT_____   HEIGHT_____

COAT LENGTH _____

IDENTIFYING MARKS_____

TYPE AND COLOR OF COLLAR _____

LICENSE#_____   RABIES TAG#_____

AREA LOST _____

DATE LOST _____

DOG'S NAME _____

OWNER'S NAME_____

ADDRESS _____

HOME PHONE_____   WORK PHONE_____

<u>ATTACH PICTURE HERE</u>

MEDICAL HEALTH RECORD

Owner's Name _____

Address _____

_____

Home Phone_____ Work Phone_____

Friend/Family For Emergency Contact _____

_____

Dog's Name_____

Breed_____

Date of Birth _____

Special Diet _____

Date	Vaccination Type
_____	_____
_____	_____
_____	_____
_____	_____
_____	_____
_____	_____
_____	_____
_____	_____
_____	_____
_____	_____
_____	_____

Date	Stool Examinations & Treatment
_____	_____
_____	_____
_____	_____

Date	Medical Examination/Treatment/Weight
_____	_____
_____	_____
_____	_____
_____	_____
_____	_____
_____	_____

Emergency Numbers

    Veterinarian_____

    After-Hour Veterinarian_____

    Poison Control_____

    National Animal Poison Control Center _____

    Fire Department_____

EMERGENCY WORKSHEET

Temperature ____   Pulse ____   Respirations ____

Where is the major problem located?

____ mouth
____ eyes
____ neck
____ chest (heart and lungs)
____ abdomen
____ back
____ urinary tract
____ legs
____ skin
____ nervous system

What kind of symptoms or problems are present? List them.

_____

_____

_____

_____

How long have the symptoms been present?

____ minutes ____ hours ____ days ____ weeks

Are the symptoms becoming ____ better ____ worse ____ same?

Have these problems occurred before?

Does the dog appear to be

____ depressed
____ disoriented
____ in pain
____ incoherent
____ excitable

NORMAL VITAL SIGNS FOR DOGS

Temperature	100 to 103 degrees Fahrenheit
Pulse/Heart Rate	100 to 130 beats per minute
Respiratory Rate	20 to 24 breaths per minute

The above signs are for a normal mature dog at rest. An excited dog, or one that has been running around, will have an elevated heart rate and an elevated respiratory rate. However, elevated vital signs for a dog at rest may be a sign of infection, disease, overheating or a variety of other health problems. Low vital signs may indicate that the dog is in shock. See Problem/Condition - Shock.

PREVENTIVE HEALTH CARE

Good health care is paramount in disease prevention. The old saying "an ounce of prevention is worth a pound of cure" definitely applies to dogs. Many fatal infections can be prevented by proper health care in the form of vaccinations, dental care, and regular worm examinations. Other advances in canine medicine, some in the form of blood tests, can also be utilized to extend a dog's lifespan.

I.   **Infections that Vaccinations Prevent**

A.   Distemper – a disease, caused by a virus, that may result in fever, severe respiratory disease and digestive upsets. Usually fatal, this disease may result in permanent neurological problems for dogs that survive.

B.   Adenovirus – a disease that may cause respiratory problems or hepatitis (inflammation of the liver).

C.   Parainfluenza – a virus that causes respiratory problems.

D.   Leptospirosis – a bacterial infection which may result in internal bleeding, digestive upsets, fever and kidney damage.

E.   Parvovirus – a highly infectious digestive infection that causes vomiting and severe bloody diarrhea. If not treated, it is usually fatal, with death occurring as soon as 24 hours after the onset of symptoms.

F.   Coronavirus – a disease similar to parvovirus except that it is typically not as severe.

G.   Bordetella (kennel cough) – a bacterial infection which causes bronchitis resulting in a debilitating cough.

H.   Lyme disease – spread by ticks, this disease causes symptoms ranging from depression and loss of appetite to fever, lameness and swollen lymph nodes.

I.   Rabies – a disease, transmitted by other infected animals, that is virtually universally fatal to animals and people.

II. Heartworm Disease

A. Heartworm disease is a contagious parasite (worm) that is spread by mosquitoes. A mosquito bites a dog and deposits, under the skin, larvae which migrate to the heart. Once they are in the heart, the larvae mature into long spaghetti-like worms that interfere with the heart and also cause lung problems.

B. There is no vaccine for heartworm, but there is preventive medication. All dogs that live in heartworm areas should be tested annually and given preventive medication.

III. Puppy Vaccinations and Care

A. Puppies should be given their first vaccinations at 6 weeks of age for distemper, adenovirus, parainfluenza, leptospirosis, parvovirus and coronavirus. These vaccinations should be repeated at 9 weeks, 12 weeks and 15 weeks of age.

B. An additional parvovirus booster vaccination should be given at 5 to 6 months of age.

C. A rabies vaccination should be given at 14 to 16 weeks of age. The rabies vaccination is given in a single shot that is effective for 1 year.

D. Protection against bordetella (kennel cough) is administered at 6 weeks of age and requires 2 vaccinations at 3 week intervals.

E. Lyme disease protection, for dogs that live in areas native to the ticks that carry the disease, requires 2 vaccines 3 weeks apart starting at age 12 weeks.

F. Heartworm protection comes in the form of a pill that the dog must take once per month. All dogs that live in regions where heartworm exists should be given this preventive medication.

G. Puppies should have a stool specimen examined under the microscope for parasites (worms, eggs and protozoa).

IV. Elective Surgery – Spaying/Neutering

A. Neutering helps prevent prostatic cancer and enlargement in male dogs.

B. Neutering prevents testicular cancer in male dogs.

C. Neutering generally improves your dog's temperament.

D. Neutering helps prevent the marking of territory with urine.

E. Altering male and female dogs will decrease roaming and running away.

F. Altering dogs prevents unwanted dog pregnancies.

G. In female dogs, the incidence of breast cancer may be decreased by having the dog spayed.

H. Both male and female dogs can usually have surgery at 5 to 6 months of age (or even earlier for some breeds). Consult your veterinarian for additional information.

V. Adult Vaccinations and Care

A. Adults not vaccinated as puppies need two vaccinations for all diseases with 3 weeks between shots, except for rabies. Rabies vaccination requires only one starting vaccine with routine booster shots every year to every 3 years.

B. Adults vaccinated as puppies need vaccination boosters every year. Rabies vaccinations may be good for 3 years depending on the type. Check with the dog's doctor.

C. Twice per year a veterinarian should check a stool specimen under the microscope for worm eggs or other parasites.

D. Every dog that lives in a heartworm region should be given a blood test once per year to check for the disease, regardless of whether the dog has been taking heartworm preventive medicine.

E. All dogs in heartworm regions should take heartworm preventive tablets. A single bite from an infected mosquito can transmit the disease.

F. A complete physical examination every year is advisable.

PHYSICAL EXAMINATION

The key to early detection of disease and health problems is knowing what to look for and how to look for it. A standard physical examination is a primary tool used by all veterinarians both to identify difficulties and to evaluate the seriousness of an emergency. By becoming familiar with the content of a physical examination, you will be able to understand your dog's symptoms better, and you will be better able to provide relevant information about your dog to your veterinarian.

I. History

As a first step in performing a physical examination, the veterinarian will ask you about the past activities of your dog. Veterinarians refer to this as a pet's history. A history helps identify numerous potential problems. For example, did the pet just return from being outside, or did a family member just treat the dog for fleas?

II. Subjective Observations (Attitude)

Next, the veterinarian will note the general attitude of the dog. Is the dog excited or depressed? Has the dog's activity level increased or decreased? Does the dog seem to be alert? Is there anything unusual about the dog's attitude or behavior?

III. Objective Observations (Physical Signs)

After the veterinarian has observed the pet's general attitude, he or she will start looking for symptoms (i.e., perform objective observations) to help pinpoint illness. The two methods veterinarians use to perform objective observations are the body system review and the spatial arrangement review.

The body system review consists of evaluating the pet's health according to the different functions of the body. The body systems include the digestive tract, urogenital system (urinary and reproductive

291

tracts), nervous system, integument system (skin), musculoskeletal system (muscle and bone), reproductive system, cardiopulmonary system (heart and lungs) and the special senses (sight, hearing and smell).

The spatial system starts at the nose and ends at the tail. The veterinarian examines the dog's entire body looking at any and all organs, muscles, bones, etc. one body part at a time (e.g., head, chest, hind quarters). Some veterinarians use a combination of the body system and the spatial arrangement.

IV. Health Checklist/Inventory

Refer to the following tables as checklists you might use to provide information to your veterinarian concerning the health of your dog. These are the types of checklists your veterinarian will use to evaluate your pet.

A. Eyes, Ears, Nose and Throat Checklist

   ____ Are the eyes clear? Cloudy? Red?

   ____ Is there discharge coming from the eyes?

   ____ Is the dog rubbing its eyes?

   ____ Are both eyes affected?

   ____ Is one eye bigger than the other?

   ____ Are the eyes moving back and forth when the dog is at rest?

   ____ Is the head tilted?

   ____ Is there any discharge coming from the ears?

   ____ Are the ear flaps swollen?

   ____ Is there discharge coming from the nose?

   ____ If there is nasal discharge, is it from both nostrils?

   ____ If there is nasal discharge, is it bloody, clear, or cloudy?

   ____ Are the gums pink? If not, what color are they? Blue? White?

   ____ Are there diseased teeth in the mouth?

   ____ Is the dog pawing at its mouth?

   ____ Is the dog drooling?

   ____ Is there blood in the dog's mouth?

B. Heart and Lungs (Cardiopulmonary) Checklist

Symptoms that may denote problems with the heart and lungs include coughing, difficult breathing, panting, fainting, collapse, blue gums, enlarged abdomen, and wheezing. Some emergency situations involving the cardiopulmonary system include heart failure, asthma, trauma (physical injury), infections and cancers. It is interesting to note that sneezing is usually associated with upper respiratory illness whereas coughing is usually associated with lower respiratory tract disorders. If you identify any of these problems, answer the following questions:

____ Is the dog coughing? Is the cough dry or productive (i.e., producing mucus)?

____ Is the dog having difficulty breathing? Does the dog's abdomen move and heave when the pet breathes?

____ Does the dog's abdomen appear enlarged?

____ Has the dog fainted or collapsed?

____ Is the dog wheezing?

____ How long have the symptoms been present?

____ How long do these spells last?

C. Digestive Tract Checklist

Your dog's appetite should be monitored. Dogs that have food available 24 hours per day pose a challenge because it is difficult to ascertain when and how much they are eating. If you feed your dog at specified times and remove any uneaten food between meals, it will be easier to monitor your dog's appetite.

Make sure your dog is fed at least twice per day. Some dogs with sensitive stomachs may need to have food available on a continuous basis, but in that case it may be possible to monitor their appetite by having dry food always available but providing canned food only once or twice per day.

Digestive symptoms include vomiting, diarrhea, painful abdomen, distended abdomen, constipation, loss of appetite, and increased digestive noises. Common digestive tract problems include

293

food poisoning, pancreatitis, cancers, foreign objects, toxins, parasites, electrolyte imbalances, kidney disease and liver disease. To help identify any of these problems, answer the following questions:

____ Has the dog been vomiting? If so, does the food look digested?

____ Is the pet eating? Has its appetite increased or decreased?

____ Is the dog eating only favorite foods?

____ How long has it been since the last meal?

____ Are the bowel movements normal? Soft? Watery? Dry?

____ Is there mucous or blood present in the dog's stool?

____ Are the dog's stools black or clay colored?

____ Is the dog constipated? How long has it been since the last bowel movement?

D. Urinary and Reproductive Tract Checklist

The most serious urinary tract problem is blockage. When a dog urinates in the house, it is important to rule out medical causes before blaming the dog for a behavioral problem. Early symptoms of blockage include straining during urination, urinating inside the house, crying while trying to urinate and severe depression. Frequent urinations and blood in the urine may also be signs of an impending medical emergency. Common reproductive and urinary tract problems include cystitis (inflamed bladder), urinary tract blockage, uterus infections, bladder stones, ruptured bladder from trauma, kidney disease and cancers. To help identify any of these problems, answer the following questions:

____ Is the dog urinating more frequently or less frequently?

____ Is the dog straining to urinate?

____ Is the dog urinating inside the house?

____ Does the dog cry when trying to urinate?

____ Is the dog urinating less volume or more volume than usual?

____ Is the dog drinking more water than usual?

____ Is the dog persistently licking its genital area?

____ Is there any discharge coming from the dog's genital area?

E. Integument (Skin) Checklist

Skin problems can arise from a multitude of causes including external parasites, burns, frostbite, lacerations and abrasions, allergies, nervous/emotional disorders and growths (benign or malignant). To help identify any skin difficulties, use the following checklist:

____ Are there any hairless areas on the dog? If so, are these areas irritated?

____ Is the dog scratching continuously?

____ Are there any lumps on the skin? If so, what size?

____ Are there any punctures or lacerations?

____ Is there any evidence of fleas or other external parasites?

____ Is there any evidence of a rash anywhere on the dog's body? If so, where is the rash?

F. Musculoskeletal (Muscle and Bone) & Nervous System Checklist

Some emergencies involving these systems include trauma, fractures, torn ligaments, disc disease, vestibular (inner ear) problems, and infections.

____ Can the dog move?

____ Is the dog limping? If so, which leg?

____ Is the dog stumbling?

____ Is the dog dragging its legs?

____ Is the dog mentally alert?

____ Does the dog walk in circles?

____ Is the dog uncoordinated?

BIBLIOGRAPHY

Alber, John I., and Delores M. Alber. *Baby-Safe Houseplants & Cut Flowers.* Highland, IL: Genus Books, 1991.

Arthurs, Kathryn, ed. *How to Grow House Plants.* 2nd ed. Menlo Park: Lane Publishing, 1974.

Davis, Lloyd E., *Handbook of Small Animal Therapeutics.* Livingston, NY: Churchill, 1985.

Fenner, William R., D.V.M., ed. *Quick Reference to Veterinary Medicine.* 2nd ed. Philadelphia: J. P. Lippincott, 1991.

Florists' Transworld Delivery Association. *Professional Guide to Green Plants.* Florists' Transworld Delivery Association, 1976.

Fowler, Murray E., D.V.M. *Plant Poisoning in Small Companion Animals.* St. Louis: Ralston Purina, 1981.

Fraser, Clarence M., ed. *The Merck Veterinary Manual.* 6th, 7th eds. Rathway, NJ: Merck & Co., 1986, 1991.

Hoskins, Johnny D. *Veterinary Pediatrics: Dogs and Cats from Birth to Six Months.* Philadelphia: W. B. Saunders, 1990.

Kirk, Robert W., D.V.M., and Stephen I. Bister, D.V.M. *Handbook of Veterinary Procedures and Emergency Treatment.* 4th ed. Philadelphia: W. B. Saunders, 1985.

Levy, Charles Kingsley, and Richard B. Primack. *A Field Guide to Poisonous Plants and Mushrooms of North America.* Brattleboro, VT: The Stephen Greene Press, 1984.

Muller, George H., Robert W. Kirk, and Danny W. Scott. *Small Animal Dermatology.* 3rd ed. Philadelphia: W. B. Saunders, 1983.

National Animal Poison Control Center. *Household Plant List.* Urbana: University of Illinois College of Veterinary Medicine.

Osweiler, Gary D., D.V. M., Thomas L. Carson, D.V.M., William B. Buck, D.V.M., and Gary A. VanGelder, D.V.M. *Clinical and Diagnostic Veterinary Toxicology.* 3rd ed. Dubuque, IA: Kendell/Hunt, 1985.

Random House Webster's College Dictionary. New York: Random House, 1991.

Taylor, Norman. *Taylor's Guide to Perennials.* Ed. Gordon P. DeWolf. Boston: Houghton Mifflin, 1961.

Tuckington, Carol. *The Home Health Guide to Poisons and Antidotes.* New York: Facts on File, 1994.

Woodward, Lucia. *Poisonous Plants: A Color Field Guide.* New York: Hippocrene Books, 1985.

INDEX

in ears, 106
in eyes, 88
DEET, 183. *See* poisoning general procedures, 182
Dehydration
and burns, 71
and diarrhea, 262
and skin irritations, 261
Deliveries of puppies, 272-274, *illus.* 274
Dental care, importance of, 257
Dental disease, 257
Dental floss, 14
Depression, 179
See also poisonous plants
Dermatitis, acute moist, 102-103
Detergents, 183. *See* poisoning general procedures, 182
Devil's ivy. *See* philodendron, 224
Diabetes, 31, 122
and collapse, 158-159
Diarrhea, 82-83, 161-162, 262-263
and acetaminophen ingestion, 54
and antifreeze ingestion, 60
and arsenic poisoning, 243
and chocolate ingestion, 73
and heat stroke, 97
and insect ingestion, 107
and intestinal parasites, 264
and uterus infection, 142
and yard chemicals, 145
bloody, 221, 231
foul-smelling, 80, 114
watery and bloody, 80, 114
See also poisonous plants
Diesel fuel, 250
Dietary changes and vomiting, 143
Digestive upset, 84-85
and flea products, 247
and ibuprofen ingestion, 105
and lead poisoning, 249
and snake bite, 132
See also poisonous plants

Digitalis. *See* foxglove, 206
Discharge
bloody, around collar, 137
cloudy, thick, from penis sheath, 116, 170
foul, under tail, 57, 142
from bite wound, 148
from vulvar area, 273
in ears, 106
Diseases
autoimmune and anemia, 59
becoming emergencies, general information, 256
cancers, 259
chronic, 260
contagious. *See* coronavirus, 80; parvovirus, 114
dental, 257
diarrhea, 262
fever, 258
infections, 258
long-term illnesses, 260
preexisting and emergency treatment, 31
skin irritations, 261
soft stools, 262
vaccinations for, 288-289
Disembowelment, 163
Dishwasher soap, 239
Disinfectants
as poisons, 239
use of. *See* wound care, 36
Dislocations, 167
Disorientation
and flea products, 247
and head tilt, 166
and inner ear disease, 106
and insect ingestion, 107
and paralysis, 111
and poisonous plants, 195, 213, 233
and shock, 124
and smoke inhalation, 129